D1560126

Aesthetic Dentistry

Quintessentials of Dental Practice – 19
Operative Dentistry - 2

Aesthetic Dentistry

By
David Bartlett
Paul A Brunton

Editor-in-Chief: Nairn H F Wilson
Editor Operative Dentistry: Paul A Brunton

Quintessence Publishing Co. Ltd.

London, Berlin, Chicago, Paris, Milan, Barcelona, Istanbul
São Paulo, Tokyo, New Delhi, Moscow, Prague, Warsaw

British Library Cataloguing-in Publication Data

Bartlett, David
  Aesthetic dentistry - (Quintessentials of dental practice;
  19. Operative dentistry; 2)
  1. Dentistry - Aesthetic aspects
  I. Title II. Brunton, Paul A. III. Wilson, Nairn H. F.
  617.6

ISBN 1850970777

ISBN 1-85097-077-7

Foreword

Aesthetic dentistry continues to grow exponentially in modern clinical practice. Patients now expect and greatly value dental attractiveness as one of the principal outcomes of routine dental care. Realising this goal can, however, be challenging. Enhancing a pleasing smile, let alone the successful management of unsightly teeth, by means that will withstand the rigours of the oral environment, demands skilful application of the art and science of both traditional and state-of-the-art dentistry, underpinned by knowledge and understanding of the many varied factors that influence the appearance of teeth individually and collectively. This is the complex subject area addressed in this excellent addition to the *Quintessentials of Dental Practice* series.

In common with all the other books in the series, *Aesthetic Dentistry* focuses on the essence of the subject matter, with high-quality illustrations distributed liberally throughout the text to highlight principles, key points, critical techniques and common pitfalls. Given the importance aesthetic dentistry has now assumed in present-day clinical practice, which is no longer limited to the three "Rs" — "repair, removal and replacement" — the information and guidance included in this book should be viewed as fundamental to the everyday business of dentistry.

As with most things in the clinical practice of dentistry, good clinical outcomes are down to trust and understanding between dentist and patient, effective communication, up-to-date knowledge, careful planning and meticulous detail in the execution of operative procedures. Good aesthetic dentistry is not easy; it is typically very demanding. This book provides a most valuable aid to meeting these demands — an excellent investment for practitioners and students with patients who would welcome an improvement in their dental appearance.

Nairn Wilson
Editor-in-Chief

Preface

This book is not meant to be a definitive textbook on aesthetic dentistry. There are already several comprehensive texts available on the subject. This book, by way of contrast, is designed to be an aide-mémoire for success, providing tips and hints for practitioners to improve their practice of everyday aesthetic techniques, coupled with a description of the underlying theory. The text will not consider single-unit indirect restorations other than certain aspects from an aesthetic point of view. Readers are referred to a specific text that considers indirect restorations in some detail. In addition, an appendix is included, which lists materials and instruments the authors have found useful.

On reading this book the reader will be able to:
- appreciate the composition and variations in the smile
- understand the theory of colour and how this affects shade-taking and colour communication
- select suitable cases for vital and non-vital bleaching
- consider the use of microabrasion to remove unsightly or unaesthetic surface defects
- apply resin composites for successful anterior laminate restorations
- prescribe successfully porcelain laminate veneers
- understand how technical, laboratory and periodontal factors can affect aesthetics
- minimise aesthetic compromises
- solve common aesthetic dilemmas.

David Bartlett
Paul A Brunton
London and Manchester, March 2005

Acknowledgements

The authors would like to thank Dr David Ricketts for reviewing and providing valuable feedback for the entire manuscript and Miss Selina Priestley for reviewing Chapter 2.

The authors are also indebted to the following individuals who have generously provided illustrations, which made the publication of this book possible: Miss Leean Morrow for the use of Figs 1-6 to 1-7 and 7-6; David Leedham for the use of Figs 2-7 to 2-9; and Tim Horwood for the use of Figs 4-5, 4-6, 5-5 and 6-5. Figs 6-4, 6-6 and 7-3 are reproduced from Dental Update by permission of George Warman Publications (UK) Ltd. Fig 6-1 is reproduced by permission of the *British Dental Journal*.

Contents

Chapter 1
Smile Dimensions

Aim

To practise successful aesthetic dentistry it is important to be familiar with the essential components of an "ideal" smile – remembering of course that the "ideal" smile is a concept around which all patient treatment is based and that every patient requires an individual approach. The aim of this chapter is to acquaint practitioners with the dimensions and components of an "ideal" smile.

Outcome

On reading this chapter practitioners will be able to assess the shape and inter-relationship of crowns and restorations within the framework of a patient's individual smile.

Introduction

Aesthetics can be viewed at two levels – the conversational and tooth levels. The conversational level considers the arrangement of teeth within the framework of a face and an individual's smile. The tooth level is the consideration of everything that makes a tooth look like a tooth. It is important that teeth should look like teeth, but equally it is important that teeth are appropriately framed. To do this effectively a practitioner must be familiar with the dimensions of a smile, to include consideration of the following:
• tooth size
• the golden proportion
• gingival position
• black triangles
• lip line
• masking gingival tissues
• moral issues.

Tooth Size

On average, the width of an upper incisor tooth is 75% of its length and

1

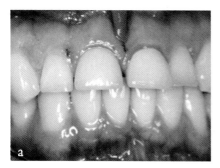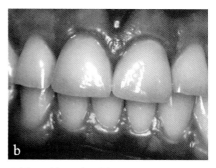

Fig 1-1 (a) Unaesthetic crowns where the width and length of the crowns are equal. (b) Replacement crown of appropriate dimensions.

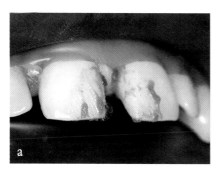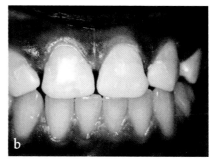

Fig 1-2 (a) Etch placed to reduce a diastema with resin composite in a young patient. (b) Post-treatment reduced diastema.

where this is not the case the result is generally unaesthetic (Fig 1-1). The perception of tooth shape, however, is very personal. For instance, someone with narrow teeth and diastemas might be quite content with their appearance. But if the patient found the appearance unacceptable and new crowns were planned for the upper incisors, it may be worthwhile to consider using this rule (width based on 75% of length) to calculate tooth width. Before any changes to width and length are embarked upon, it is essential that a diagnostic wax–up is used to assess the proposed changes to a patient's appearance. If necessary, directly placed resin composites can be used either for the short or medium term to assess the final appearance of the teeth before proceeding to the definitive treatment (Fig 1-2). The aesthetics of present-day resin composite often make the definitive stage of treatment unnecessary.

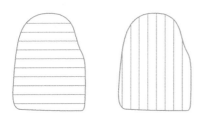

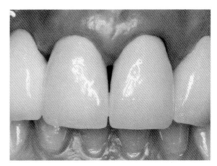

Fig 1-3 Horizontal lines make the identical crown appear shorter than the crown with the vertical lines.

Fig 1-4 A rounded or smooth contact region can make the crown appear broader, but for one that is too broad making a more pronounced angle just away from the contact point creates the illusion of a narrower crown.

The width-to-length ratio influences the judgement to close diastemas. If the ratio of the tooth is above 75% then widening the tooth further to reduce the space may produce an appearance that is unacceptable. The compromise and closure might be acceptable for a narrow tooth that could easily be widened, but for a broader tooth other factors may need to be considered. In such cases the location of the gingival tissues down the length of the crown is another assessment that is important.

Traditionally, some clinicians have linked tooth shape with gender. Narrower teeth may be found in females, broader ones in males. This demarcation is by no means accurate, and when bridgework or indirect restorations are planned clinicians normally have the advantage of other standing teeth to guide decisions on the shape and contour of the restoration. There are various technical tricks that can be adopted to hide or attenuate the angles of laboratory-made crowns. Mid-line horizontal lines appear to shorten the crown, while vertical ones nearer the proximal angles would broaden it (Fig 1-3). Additionally, if the space is too wide an illusion can be created by introducing sharp angles away from the proximal surface to make the crown appear narrower (Fig 1-4).

The most important criterion in making a judgement on aesthetics is the patient. The perceptions of colour and shape are somewhat age-related. Senior patients commonly perceive bigger and brighter teeth as indicative of youth. Unfortunately, there is an increasing trend to achieve brighter and whiter teeth producing shades that are lighter than B1. The result for many practitioners is too artificial, but increasingly patients expect and demand shades at this end of the spectrum. If such a shade is contemplated, considerable discussion should occur preoperatively and the patient should be given a clear idea what the shade is likely to look like within the parameters of their individual smile.

The Golden Proportion

Normally lateral incisors are smaller than centrals, and if their comparative size starts to become equal the result can be aesthetically unacceptable. The golden proportion adopts this concept with a balance between the canines, laterals and central incisors. The golden proportion was formulated as one of Euclid's elements *c.* 300 BC and it applies to dental aesthetics. This is amply illustrated by the fact that the central incisors are in golden proportion to the lateral incisors, which in turn are in golden proportion to the canines (Fig 1-5). Put simply, the central incisor is 1.618 wider than the lateral incisor. It is possible using grids that are based on the width of the central incisor to determine the width of a patient's smile. It is important to recognise that the proportion of the smaller to the greater – for example, the width of the central incisor in relation to the width of the lateral incisor – is golden but so also is the width of the central incisor in relation to the combined widths of the two teeth. It is accepted that when teeth are set up so that the proportion is golden within the confines of the smile it is aesthetically pleasing.

The width of a patient's smile is in golden proportion to the rest of the face. Upon smiling the anterior aesthetic segment is framed by the lips and there is space between the teeth and the corners of the mouth. This neutral space is all too often filled with over-contoured teeth or dental arches that have been made too wide. If this neutral space is lost the smile is not aesthetically pleasing. The width of the anterior aesthetic segment is in golden proportion to the width of the smile, ideally with the midline coincidental with the midline of the face.

Gingival Position

The gingival position on the upper lateral incisors in a healthy state is closer to the occlusal plane than on the central incisors and canines. Either naturally, or as a result of tooth wear and dentoalveolar compensation, this position may alter and result in the lateral incisors having a similar height to the incisors. The unworn step effect produces a natural and pleasing

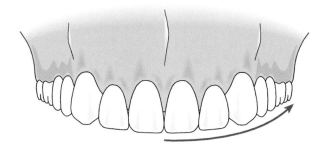

Fig 1-5 Teeth in golden proportion.

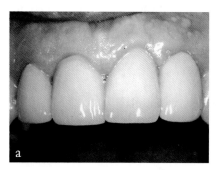
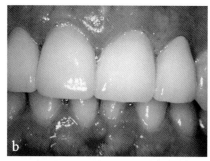

Fig 1-6 (a) Unaesthetic crowns with unequal gingival heights and teeth in incorrect proportion to each other. (b) New crowns provided for the patient after crown lengthening surgery.

appearance and can accentuate the dominance of the upper central incisors, providing an acceptable aesthetic result (Fig 1-6). Whether it is acceptable to undertake crown lengthening surgery to produce this step height appearance is doubtful but if, for instance, surgery was planned as part of the treatment for tooth wear, placing this step in the gingival position is worth considering.

The location of the gingival margin needs to be symmetrical. Unilateral gingival recession may not create a clinical problem if the patient has a low lip line. But in someone with a high lip line, unequal gingival contours may compromise the appearance of the anterior teeth (Fig 1-7). Surgical procedures aimed at adjusting the gingival position are, however, outside the remit

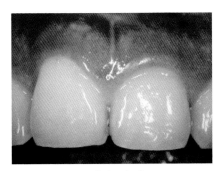 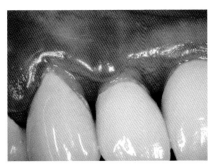

Fig 1-7 Unequal gingival contours.

Fig 1-8 Recession post root planing, showing ill-fitting crowns placed with subgingival margins.

of this book and readers are referred to a specialist textbook in periodontics. This problem, however, should be considered at the treatment-planning stage and help sought from a periodontist, if appropriate.

Perhaps the most avoidable periodontal problem is where the gingival margin of the preparation is placed. Placing preparation margins too subgingivally will result in a long-term periodontal problem. This is especially the case if the patient is susceptible to periodontal disease, as this might well result in gingival recession, thereby exposing margins that had previously been placed within the gingival crevice (Fig 1-8). One area of the preparation most commonly affected by this is the interdental region. Cutting through the interdental papilla is quite common and, while this may not make the impression-taking too difficult, it might result in the labial gingival margin becoming unstable. If the patient is susceptible to periodontal disease then this will cause localised recession in the interdental area, but unfortunately this change will result in an unstable gingival margin labially too and as a result the gingival position may change quite quickly. Therefore the most appropriate position for the margin is just within the gingival sulcus, sufficient to hide the margin but not to encourage gingival inflammation. When positioning the margins of preparations, bear in mind that only 33% of the population show the gingival third of their teeth when they smile (Fig 1-9). Juxtagingival preparation margins would be appropriate with this group of patients.

Black Triangles

For many practitioners and patients the appearance of the black triangle

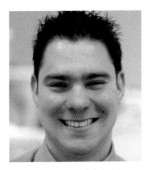 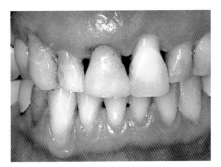

Fig 1-9 Gingival third is not visible when most people smile.

Fig 1-10 Black triangles post periodontal disease.

between teeth is unacceptable, as it is associated with ageing (Fig 1-10). It is, however, difficult to overcome. If the tooth is narrow then broadening the crown with direct resin composites, porcelain veneers or crowns may hide some of the black area. It is important, however, to assess the original width of the crown before this is contemplated. It is not sensible to widen a tooth that is already too broad, whereas with a narrow tooth a degree of change can be contemplated. Another important assessment is the location of the adjacent gingival margins:

- If a ratio of around 75–85% of length to width is possible the tooth can be widened to bulk out the gingival tissues and so hide the triangle. If the result is still not predictable, even with a diagnostic wax-up, direct resin composite build-ups can be used either provisionally or for the medium term to assess changes to the width of teeth. For simplicity, a resin reinforced glass ionomer or a low-viscosity resin composite without etching and a bonding agent can be added to the tooth to alter the shape. When needed the material can then be simply removed.

- Assess the proximal height of the gingival tissues of the teeth to be prepared. If the recession is a localised phenomenon it might be possible to relocate tissues occlusally to reduce the impact of the interdental area; however, the stability of the result is questionable. If the recession is more generalised, relocation of the periodontal tissues is less likely to be successful.

- It is important to determine the position of the cementoenamel junction. If the margin is below the gingival margin then some degree of flexibility may be possible in relocating the tissues in an apical direction. If the periodontal tissues are significantly below the cementoenamel junction then this would not be possible.

- It may be possible to consider orthodontic movement to intrude or extrude the tooth to move its relationship with the other teeth. The stability of such movements needs careful consideration and may require to be accompanied by modification of tooth shape to maintain occlusal stability.
- In cases in which teeth are missing, such as implant-supported bridges, the pontic can be overbuilt to create an acceptable gingival contour. These so-called ovate pontics can be quite successful.

Lip Line

In a typical smile about a third of the upper incisors are visible in patients with Class I or II incisal relationships during normal function, and this display is pleasing. In patients with a Class III incisal relationship, where the lower incisors are more prominent, this appearance is generally not attainable.

Different problems start to develop when the patient displays too much of the teeth – for instance, someone with a high lip line. The aesthetic demands in such cases are much greater. Wherever the margins of the restorations are placed they will eventually become visible. This is because, in time, even with the best periodontal health at baseline, there will be some gingival recession. As the gingival tissues migrate apically the margin of the restoration will become more visible. On darkened root-filled teeth this appearance can be unsightly, but is difficult to change. If the tooth is then reprepared by cutting away more dentine apically, the crown of the tooth becomes longer and may become too narrow. This can also weaken the tooth, let alone affect the subsequent vitality of the teeth. Some changes to the position of the gingivae may be possible with periodontal surgery but the result may not be stable, particularly in the long term. For teeth that have very long clinical crowns masking procedures need to be considered.

Masking Gingival Tissues

This is perhaps one of the most difficult clinical problems for practitioners. In a healthy mouth loss of localised gingival tissues may be treated by means of grafting. How stable the result is will vary from patient to patient and their ability to maintain their oral hygiene is an important consideration. However, when relocation surgery is not possible alternatives are necessary, and unfortunately they are all compromises. The most effective soft-tissue replacement is acrylic, which is thinned at the edges and made to merge in with the adjacent tissues (Fig 1-11). Pink porcelain can be added to the gingival surfaces of crowns to mimic the gingival tissues but is only really effec-

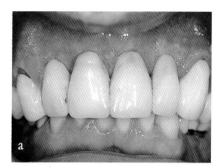 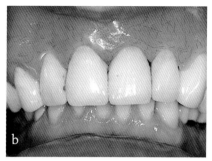

Fig 1-11 (a) Gingival recession. (b) Same patient with a gingival mask in place.

tive in very small additions. An important consideration is the bulk of the porcelain needed. With too much it will be difficult to control the cooling of the porcelain after firing, and the bulk of porcelain may fracture. The most difficult situation is considerable recession with a high lip line. In these situations removable acrylic gingival masks have been suggested, but these are inconvenient for patients as they have to be removed regularly for cleaning, let alone plaque accumulation, which may cause more gingival recession.

Moral Issues

Although the "ideal smile" may for some be an appropriate choice, for others it could be considered over-treatment. So it is essential to strike the appropriate balance. Comprehensive treatment planning involves listening to the patient and understanding their needs in combination with consideration of possibilities of the techniques available, cost of treatment and a practitioner's clinical skill. Some practitioners are using photo-manipulation to show patients the anticipated result of a clinical treatment. While this can be helpful it should be remembered that the end result clinically is never as predictable as the manipulated image, and it may be unwise for patients to have raised expectations for a treatment. A diagnostic wax-up can provide a helpful preoperative guide to the end result without increasing the expectations too much, but as a tool it is somewhat crude. Using photographs of patients when they were younger can also be helpful, but unfortunately no dentistry can reverse the ageing process.

Whichever treatment is chosen, the patient needs fully to understand the treatment concepts and choices. To do this a letter describing the planned outcomes and the choices is mandatory. It is sensible not to choose the options at the first visit. This is especially true for more complicated procedures. Never forget to document everything and, where possible, take clinical photographs, not only to help with the diagnosis but also as a record of treatment.

Further Reading

Levin EI. Dental aesthetics and the golden proportion. J Prosthet Dent 1978;40:244-252.

Chapter 2
Shade and Colour

Aim

Successful shade-taking and colour communication are sources of great difficulty for practitioners. The aim of this chapter is to improve understanding of modern methods of shade-taking and colour communication. The importance of shape and form in successful aesthetics will also be outlined.

Outcome

Practitioners will understand the basics of colour theory, be familiar with how to take a shade effectively and understand how shape and form can impact on aesthetic dentistry.

Introduction

Colour can be described as having three components — hue, chroma and value — which are defined as follows:
- Hue - type of colour (for example, red, green, blue).
- Chroma - depth or saturation of the hue (for example, pink).
- Value - brightness of the hue (for example, grey or whiteness).

The components can be classified on a three-dimensional (3D) scale called a colour sphere. The X, Y and Z axes meet at various points to produce a colour. In clinical practice colour is an important consideration when choosing the shade for tooth-coloured restorations such as direct resin composites and crowns. Equally, in an individual patient the teeth may all have the same hue (colour) but the chroma (depth or saturation of the hue) may differ from one tooth to another. For example, a canine can appear yellower than a small lateral incisor in the same patient's mouth. The underlying colour may be the same, but in the canine the thickness of enamel and dentine is greater, which gives a darker colour (Fig 2-1). Similarly the shade of a tooth varies within the tooth in that the neck usually appears darker than the tip. Teeth, for the same reasons, become darker the further back they are in the dental arch. For example, lateral incisors appear darker than central incisors

11

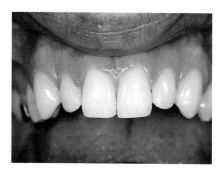

Fig 2-1 Canines are darker than the incisors.

because the thickness of the enamel is much reduced, especially in the cervical area. Consequently the underlying dentine, which is largely responsible for the colour of a tooth, comes to the fore.

Colour changes also occur as a result of tooth wear. As a tooth is affected by abrasion, attrition or erosion, either in isolation or in combination, the thickness of the remaining enamel and dentine gradually reduces. The colour saturation or chroma changes as the effect of the colour of the underlying dentine again becomes more dominant. Often teeth are described as becoming more yellow with age. They are not in fact more yellow, they just appear so as the underlying dentine becomes more opaque (less translucent) through age-related sclerosis and the modifying effects of the overlying enamel.

Enamel is more translucent than dentine. This is often very apparent in young people who frequently have translucent incisal edges. To complicate matters further the overlying enamel has variable thickness. As the patient ages this translucency is lost as the tooth wears and the incisal tip reduces. This has various consequences. For example, over the labial face of a tooth different shades are typically present. A tooth is unlikely to be a single shade – for example, towards the incisal tip the colour of A2 is a lighter blue while at the gingival margin a darker red. The incisal translucency frequently represents the relative absence of dentine, while at the gingival margin there will be some reflection of the periodontal tissues.

Shade-Matching

To help match crowns to natural teeth most manufacturers of porcelains and resin composites produce shade guides. The most commonly used guide is the Vita Classic shade guide (VITA Zahnfabrik H. Rauter GmbH

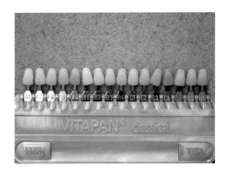

Fig 2-2 Vita Classic shade guide.

& Co. KG, D-79713 Bad Säckingen, Germany), which has almost universal acceptance (Fig 2-2). Many manufacturers have produced better-designed guides, but nothing seems to have replaced the original Vita Classic shade guide. The guide is divided into reddish brown (A), reddish yellow (B), grey (C) and reddish grey (D) shades. There are two main hues in the A and B shade guide tabs. The C and D tabs represent lower values of B and A tabs, respectively. In most circumstances the shade guide provides a sufficiently wide spectrum of choice to map most people's teeth.

The Vita Classic shade guide makes the operator think about hue. For example, the patient's teeth are matched to an A hue and then, using the Vita Classic shade guide, the shade is selected from A1, A2, A3, A3.5 or A4. In contrast, the new Vita 3D master shade guide, which clusters hues of similar value, makes the operator think about value first and chroma second and is arguably superior in this respect (Fig 2-3). A more accurate method might include the laboratory providing a custom-made shade guide for each tooth made by the technician supporting the practitioner.

Tips for Choosing the Right Shade
- Colour is NOT the most important factor when selecting the correct shade for a restoration, and it should not be the first consideration.

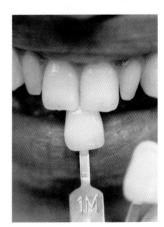

Fig 2-3 Master shade guide in 3D.

- Look at the patient's skin tone.
- Look initially at the adjacent teeth.
- Consider the surface anatomy, concentrating on shape, form, texture and contour. The eye perceives shape before shade, so it is important to get the shape, texture and contour right at the start. Arguably, a restoration that is correctly shaped and formed but a shade out will pass, while a correctly shaded but poorly contoured restoration will not.
- Draw a diagram on the laboratory sheet to assist the technician. Include surface characteristics such as cracks, surface-staining, areas of opalescence and other surface topography you wish to include (Fig 2-4). The texture of the surface of the tooth can have a profound effect on the perceived shade, and for this reason a biscuit bake try-in of a metal ceramic crown is not very helpful for assessing its final appearance.
- Remember to include the age and gender of the patient on the laboratory prescription form, as this information is very helpful for the technician.
- Colour photographs are useful for communicating the surface characteristics of the tooth to the laboratory and, to a certain degree, with shade assessment. Although many practitioners will have the facilities for colour photography, black-and-white photography can also be very useful, in particular in difficult cases. Black-and-white photographs are particularly helpful in assisting the technician to assess the correct value, provided the photograph is taken under good lighting conditions.
- To assess the shade of the tooth it is helpful to arrange the shade guide according to value running from the lightest to the darkest — say, from B1 to C4 (Fig 2-5). Alternatively, first choose the hue and then the chroma. For example, the hue may be A and then the choice is A1, A2, A3, A3.5 or A4.
- In general, the older the patient the darker the tooth. Consequently be wary of choosing very light shades, such as A1, for a 50-year-old; generally the teeth of mature adults have a chroma of 3 or 3.5.

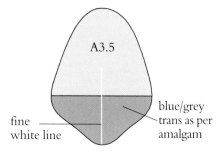

Fig 2-4 Laboratory prescription.

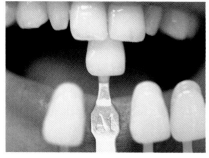

Fig 2-5 Vita Classic shade guide arranged according to value.

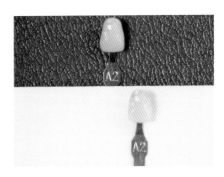

Fig 2-6 The effect of background on shade perception. These shades are actually the same but one appears darker.

- There is trend toward lighter shades, with many A1 and A2 being selected. This is almost certainly as a consequence of large numbers of patients having had some form of dental bleaching coupled with patient requests for lighter teeth.
- Always take the shade with the patient either sitting or standing, never supine. This is because it is sensible to assess shade under similar conditions, in terms of lighting, as the restoration will ultimately be viewed. If a shade is taken with the patient in a supine position, the lighting conditions are completely different. This will affect both shade determination and in turn the aesthetic acceptability of the restoration.
- Hold the guide at arm's length, adjacent to the tooth surface. Move the guide from tooth to tooth taking care not to stare too long. Periodically ask the patient to moisten the teeth with saliva.
- Take short sharp glimpses at the teeth. Glance at the teeth then look away. This is to minimise the effects of fatigue of rods and cones in the operator's eyes.
- Be aware of contrast enhancement, given that the background can have an effect on the perceived shade. For example, a shade will look different on white and black backgrounds (Fig 2-6). To assist in shade-taking, always have the tab in the same vertical plane as the tooth you are matching and ask the patient to posture their tongue forward to give a consistent and meaningful (tissue-coloured) background against which to take the shade.
- Light plays a critical role in assessing colour, remembering that colour is primarily a function of the available light. Try and use natural daylight that is not too bright when selecting a shade. Very bright natural daylight may result in the selection of too light a shade. If the surgery has a window, it is helpful to have the patient stand by the window when taking a shade.
- If natural light is not possible, use a natural light lamp. Alternatively, make sure the fluorescent lights in the surgery are colour- corrected. Ideally, the

lighting source you use should be the same as the one the technician uses in the laboratory to produce the restoration. It is sensible, therefore, to ascertain that your laboratory has the same colour-corrected tubes. Colour-corrected tubes, however, are only part of the answer as they can be somewhat variable.

- The effects of metamarism, which occurs when the colour of an object – a tooth, for example – appears different in different lighting conditions, should be minimised. To do this, try and assess the shade in at least two different lighting conditions. For example, assess the shade in both surgery and daylight or, if daylight is not available, try assessing the shade in dimmed and bright surgery lighting conditions.
- Your first decision is normally correct. Experience suggests that the longer it takes to assess the shade the more likely it is that the shade is incorrect.
- If a patient has a shade in the C or D ranges check again. They are relatively uncommon shades in natural teeth.
- It is helpful to ask your nurse's opinion and wise to include the patient in the final decision.
- Another option is to involve the technician in shade selection.

Pixels v. Rods and Cones

Recently computer technology has made significant progress into clinical dentistry. Although computers were introduced into dental surgeries primarily for data transmission, the digital revolution has seen many further applications, one of which has been the use of digital images for shade-taking and colour communication.

Computer-based shade-taking systems, an example of which is illustrated in Fig 2-7, are thought to have the advantages of controlled illumination, which

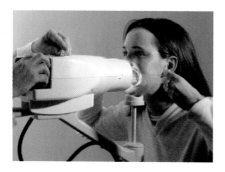

Fig 2-7 Ikam™ digital shade taking system.

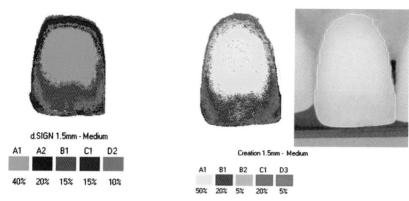

Fig 2-8 Polychromatic map.   **Fig 2-9** Digital analysis.

is reported to produce more consistent results. There are several systems on the market, some of which are useful for taking base shades, while others provide polychromatic and/or translucency maps (Figs 2-8 and 2-9). One system that has been introduced has clinical and laboratory applications. A digital image of the teeth and a grey standard is taken under two lighting conditions — natural colour-corrected light and polarised light. These images are analysed by the associated software and transmitted to the laboratory, where suggested shades are shown on a polychromatic prescription which the technician uses to build up the indirect restoration. The laboratory has a set-up similar to that used in the clinic. The restoration can be imaged and the shade analysed to ensure it matches the original prescription before it is returned to the clinician. Further research is needed to evaluate these systems before they can be recommended for routine use. The general consensus is that it is best to proceed as follows if you have a digital shade-taking system:

• Take a visual shade.
• Take a computerised digital shade and compare. If they agree you probably have the correct shade.
• Send this shade to the laboratory along with a digital image, including the two closest matching shade tabs.
• Remember that no matter how good the technology, the result is still dependent on the skill of the technician and having sufficient space in which to develop an aesthetically pleasing restoration.

Further Reading

Aoshima H. A Collection of Ceramic Works: A Communication Tool for the Dental Office and Laboratory. Berlin: Quintessenz Verlag, 1993.

Chapter 3
Bleaching and Microabrasion

Aim

Bleaching is a minimally interventionist means of improving the brightness of vital and non-vital teeth. Microabrasion is a useful (often adjunctive) technique for removing localised enamel discoloration from anterior teeth. In carefully selected cases microabrasion can be usefully combined with vital bleaching procedures to improve anterior aesthetics. The aim of this chapter is to consider different non-vital and vital bleaching procedures along with the technique of microabrasion.

Outcome

Practitioners will be familiar with the advantages, disadvantages, indications and contraindications for various methods of bleaching vital and non-vital teeth. Equally, practitioners will be familiar with the technique of microabrasion.

Introduction

The colour of teeth is very subjective. It means different things to different people. For example, a patient may be convinced that their teeth are too dark and yet to the practitioner they appear to be within the normal colour range. This commonly occurs with canines, which are wrongly described by patients as being a mismatch in colour with their anterior teeth. Canines are darker than incisors, but this is the natural result of the canine being thicker buccolingually than the other anterior teeth. Differences in the assessment of the colour of teeth between patient and clinician can be an important consideration when obtaining informed consent for bleaching procedures, as it is not possible to guarantee that the technique will be successful, let alone how long the bleaching effect will last.

Common Causes of Tooth Discoloration

The causes of tooth discoloration can be classified as follows:
Localised
Trauma:
• permanent teeth

- developing teeth.

Superficial staining:
- extrinsic causes – dietary, smoking or plaque-related
- caries
- discoloured restoration.

Generalised
Acquired:
- age-related
- tetracycline
- fluorosis.

Hereditary:
- amelogenesis imperfecta
- dentinogenesis imperfecta.

It is clear that there are a number of causes for tooth discolouration and the diagnosis is important, as this will determine how an individual case is managed.

Trauma
Damage to the blood supply of fully developed teeth may result in the loss of vitality. The pulpal tissues degenerate, sometimes acutely, producing a non-vital tooth. The blood pigments left behind following pulp degeneration include haemoglobin, which infiltrates the dentinal tubules, leading to significant tooth discoloration when this breaks down. This stain can vary in intensity from very dark to almost imperceptible. The intensity of the discoloration will in general determine the time needed to bleach the tooth and in some cases the likelihood of success.

Infrequently, trauma to a deciduous tooth will damage the developing permanent replacement. The result might be a change in colour and shape of the permanent tooth. The discoloration, provided it is not too intense, may be corrected. The change in shape may necessitate the provision of a veneer or crown in adult life.

Superficial staining
Superficial extrinsic staining can be removed by a thorough scaling and polishing. Common dietary supplements — for example, tannin — will cause a superficial stain to develop on the exposed surfaces of teeth. Smoking can also cause extensive extrinsic staining of teeth – in particular, in heavy smok-

ers. Such stains, although superficial, can be quite resistant to routine cleaning and polishing techniques. Whitening toothpastes, containing emulsifiers and titanium dioxide, may remove superficial stain and appear to whiten the teeth. They are particularly useful for removing dietary stains, tobacco tars and for shade maintenance after bleaching.

Occasionally, a chromogenic-type bacterium colonises the gingival crevice of patients with poor oral hygiene. This causes a green/black stain along the cervical margin of the teeth. Typically, a routine prophylaxis fails to remove such surface stain and either bleaching or tooth reduction is required.

Age-related changes
As people age their teeth darken or appear darker. This may be a result of the enamel wearing, exposing the underlying darker dentine, and/or the effect of age-related sclerosis of dentine: consequently the tooth appears darker. This apparent change must be balanced against the patient's age, as the actual colour change with age might not be so prominent. Equally the tooth colour may appear to be natural while lighter teeth would appear unnatural when framed by an older face.

Tetracycline
Prescribing tetracycline for non-critical infections in patients with developing teeth is now considered to be indefensible. Consequently, the incidence of tetracycline discoloration is decreasing, notably in the UK. This is in contrast to other parts of the developing world. The tetracycline molecule becomes incorporated into developing tooth tissues, changing the colour of dentine from which teeth get their inherent colour (Fig 3-1). The degree of yellow to blue-grey discoloration depends on the nature and concentration of tetracycline administered to the patient and the exposure of the tetracycline-containing tooth tissues to ultraviolet light following eruption. Some brown/yellow tetra-

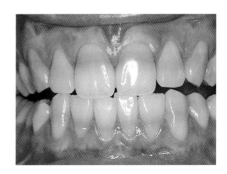

Fig 3-1 Tetracycline staining.

cycline stains are relatively easy to overcome using vital bleaching techniques. Blue-grey tetracycline stains often remain resistant to bleaching.

Fluorosis
The intake of excessive amounts of fluoride during tooth crown formation may result in brown and white speckled mottling of the tooth – fluorosis. Concentrations of more than 1ppm of fluoride in drinking water increase the risk of fluorosis – in particular if large amounts of toothpaste or other dietary supplements of fluoride are taken at the same time.

Bleaching or removing the superficial layer of enamel with microabrasion normally eliminates brown mottling. The surrounding white speckled opacity is more difficult to remove but usually responds favourably to vital bleaching. These less interventive management techniques are usually preferred to crowns or veneers, since no tooth tissue needs to be sacrificed.

Hereditary causes
Dentinogenesis imperfecta and amelogenesis imperfecta are relatively rare conditions. It can be difficult to differentiate these conditions clinically. Dentinogenesis imperfecta (hereditary opalescent dentine) is characterised by bulbous root formation and an absence of root canals. Radiographs are invaluable in confirming a diagnosis of dentinogenesis imperfecta. Amelogenesis imperfecta is more difficult to diagnose, as the condition has a variable presentation. Confusing amelogenesis imperfecta with marked fluorosis is not unusual.

Vital Bleaching

Hydrogen Peroxide (H_2O_2)
Hydrogen peroxide has been used to bleach teeth for over a century. Bleaching (lightening or brightening) teeth is an effective treatment for stained and discoloured sound teeth. Vital tooth-bleaching has the added advantages of being both less interventive and conservative of tooth tissues. Alternative treatments, such as veneers, all-ceramic crowns and metal–ceramic crowns, by necessity require extensive tooth-tissue removal. Vital tooth-bleaching, in common with most clinical procedures, is not without some risk. This risk is, however, low. Balanced against the risk of a tooth becoming non-vital after crowning, bleaching remains the initial treatment of choice to improve the appearance of discoloured teeth. Although veneers and crowns can improve the appearance of discoloured teeth, they can never reproduce the translucency and vibrancy of the intact tooth.

Mode of action

Hydrogen peroxide is a minute molecule. As a consequence, it is able to penetrate enamel and dentine, effecting a change that results in bleaching. Hydrogen peroxide, or those products that degrade to produce it, dissociates to form the superoxide ion and water. It is the high reactivity of the superoxide ion which is thought to be responsible for the bleaching process. The reactive ion removes the stains from teeth by oxidising pigments trapped in the structures of enamel and dentine. Most clinical techniques for bleaching rely on this effect but vary the speed by either extending the periods of contact, using higher concentrations or, as previously practised, heating the bleaching agent.

Carbamide Peroxide

Carbamide peroxide, otherwise known as urea peroxide, breaks down to form hydrogen peroxide and urea. In the oral environment the hydrogen peroxide forms the superoxide ion and water, while the urea forms ammonia and carbon dioxide. The amount of urea formed as part of the breakdown is too small to have any biological consequence. Most research on the safety and efficacy of carbamide peroxide has been on a 10% concentration. More recently, higher concentrations have been produced that increase the speed of reaction and so the bleaching process. A 10% solution of carbamide peroxide produces 3.35% hydrogen peroxide, a 15% solution of carbamide peroxide produces 5% hydrogen peroxide and a 35% carbamide peroxide (chair-side bleaching) gives 10% hydrogen peroxide. To avoid any adverse reactions care must be taken to use solutions and gels of carbamide peroxide according to manufacturer's directions.

Safety

In the past, bleaching has been used to lighten non-vital teeth. Only in the past 15 years or so has the bleaching of vital teeth become more common. There are risks associated with any operative procedure: using hydrogen peroxide to bleach teeth is no exception. In the early days the technique carried a relatively high risk of subsequent resorption because heat was used to activate the hydrogen peroxide. More recently, the potential for systemic effects has raised concerns, none of which has, to date, found any scientific support. The main concern with hydrogen peroxide is its potential to cause cellular damage. Most of the studies undertaken to investigate this effect have used animal models, with high concentrations per body weight applied for extended periods of time. It is difficult to extrapolate the effects of hydrogen peroxide under such situations to the clinical situation. Hydrogen peroxide is a by-product of human enzymatic action, which is then naturally degraded by enzymes to reduce its potentially damaging effect. Despite the results from animal studies suggesting toxic effects on small mammals, the likely risk to human beings is very low. The consensus of opinion based on research is that the risk of damaging side-effects from hydrogen peroxide or other associated products used to bleach vital or non-vital teeth is small. In essence, the benefits of the treatment far outweigh the theoretical risks of the procedure.

Effects on Teeth and Restorative Materials

Findings from laboratory studies suggest that bleaching has no adverse effect on tooth tissues. Studies on enamel hardness and the bond strength of resin composites to bleached enamel have failed to demonstrate any clinically significant effects of bleaching. There is less research available on the effects of bleaching on dentine bonding but the effect, as with enamel, would appear to be negligible.

When restoring bleached teeth it is generally recommended to delay the provision of restorations of resin composites or glass ionomer cements for at least 24 hours following completion of bleaching. One of the effects of bleaching is dehydration of the tooth surface. Although rehydration tends to occur quickly (<24 hours), it is advisable to be satisfied that sufficient time has elapsed before proceeding to provide tooth-coloured restorations. An alternative approach is to place restorations before bleaching, but this has the disadvantage of exposing the surfaces of recently placed restorations to hydrogen peroxide. Furthermore, it is difficult to predict shade following bleaching. A common clinical outcome of bleaching is patients requesting restorations be changed to match the new colour of the teeth. It is helpful, therefore, to warn the patients that anterior restorations may need to be replaced following bleaching.

If new crowns are placed after bleaching the adjacent teeth may gradually revert to their original pre-bleached colour and the crowns will appear too bright. Minimally prepared teeth restored with restorations of translucent porcelain – for example, resin-bonded crowns or laminate veneers – may have a slightly different response to bleaching. The bleaching material may pass through the marginal interface to affect the colour of the underlying dentine, which will, in turn, affect the colour of the restored unit. More likely, if bleached teeth are subsequently crowned or veneered, the core of the tooth may darken over time, resulting in a darkening of the restored tooth. Previous clinical experience with veneers has shown that darkening a veneered tooth can be corrected by rebleaching via the palatal surface, with an appropriately designed bleaching splint. If full-coverage crowns are prescribed post-bleaching it is prudent to use a system that has some form of coping to protect the restoration from changes in the colour of the underlying dentine.

The effects of bleaching materials on amalgams have also been investigated. It is unlikely that the bleaching agents used will result in the release of significant levels of mercury, and any mercury released is within recognised safety limits. Occasionally, amalgam restorations may change from a dark to a more silver appearance.

Stability of Bleaching

The response of vital teeth to bleaching is variable. It is not unknown for bleached teeth to remain whitened for decades. In other cases the effects may be short-lived. In most patients the colour of their bleached teeth will remain stable for periods of up to two to three years after which "top-up" bleaching may be required. If the change occurs more quickly, within months, then another bleaching technique or restorative technique is probably indicated. This problem with the stability of the treatment outcome should be balanced against the choice of other irreversible, more destructive restorative techniques, many of which may often have a similar life expectancy. Either way, the patient should be warned about the risk before starting treatment.

Preservation of Tooth Tissue

Many patients will feel comfortable with bleaching as a conservative technique and will accept this treatment over more invasive ones, such as veneers or crowns. This is especially true of younger patients once they realise that restorations may last only a few years. A restoration placed early in life will in all probability need to be replaced many times, resulting inevitably in the loss of more tooth tissue each time it is replaced. In due course repeated treatments will lead to a loss of vitality and critical weakening of the remaining tooth tissues.

The choice whether to bleach teeth or provide veneers or crowns depends on the restorative status of the teeth to be treated. Generally speaking, bleaching should be undertaken only on sound or minimally restored teeth. Teeth with extensive restorations are probably more appropriately treated with crowns.

The bleaching process lightens the teeth but not restorations. Therefore, if extensive restorations are present they will need to be replaced following bleaching. Over time bleached tooth tissue may darken but the colour of the replaced resin composites will remain stable, resulting in a colour mismatch.

Side-effects

The most common side-effect with vital bleaching is cervical sensitivity, which can have an incidence as high as 50%. In most patients this is tolerable and does not interfere with the quality of life of the patient, nor is it likely to compromise the vitality of the tooth. In others, the symptoms disappear within a few days. In cases in which the sensitivity becomes unbearable for patients treatment should be discontinued. The authors have found that concurrent use of a daily fluoride mouthwash and/or the once-only application of a dentine desensitiser, often pre-treatment, help to reduce sensitivity.

It is important to supervise the bleaching process, providing the patient with advice and support during the procedure. Some practitioners manage this by providing patients with a limited number of tubes of bleaching agent and reviewing the patient at one- or two-week intervals. Others will regularly review their patients to ensure that any problems are managed effectively and safely. It is suggested that weekly reviews during the active treatment phase are preferable.

Indications

Vital bleaching procedure is considered to be indicated for the following conditions:
• Mild generalised staining.
• Age-related yellow discoloration (Fig 3-2).
• Mild tetracycline staining.
• Very mild fluorosis.
• Acquired superficial staining.
• Tobacco staining.
• Absorptive and penetration stains (tea and coffee).
• Colour change related to pulpal trauma.
• Patients who request a non-interventive approach to the management of their tooth discoloration.
• Young patients with an inherited grey or yellow hue to their teeth.

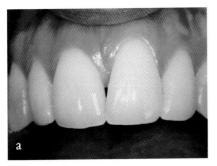 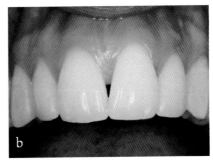

Fig 3-2 (a) Yellow discoloration. (b) After bleaching for two weeks with 10% carbamide peroxide.

Contraindications

Vital bleaching is contraindicated as follows:
- Severe tetracycline staining, pitting hypoplasia and fluorosis stain. The more intense, stains such as tetracycline or fluorosis, respond slowly and therefore require greater compliance from the patient than an age-related stain.
- Discoloration in the adolescent patient with large pulps.
- Patients with unrealistic expectations.
- Teeth with extensive, inadequate or defective restorations contraindicate the technique, as there is a possibility that the bleaching agent will penetrate tooth restoration interfaces to cause sensitivity. More appropriate techniques, such as crowns, should be used to improve the appearance of the tooth. Therefore, the technique is more suitable for sound or minimally restored teeth.
- Teeth with excessive tooth wear – in particular, erosion.
- Teeth with deep surface cracks and fracture lines.
- Teeth with apical pathology.
- Fractured teeth.
- Pregnant women or nursing mothers.
- Teeth excessively sensitive to heat, cold, touch and sweetness.
- Lack of compliance with proposed regime.

Advantages

Vital tooth-bleaching has the following advantages, which are of direct benefit to the patient:
- Conservative of tooth tissue.
- Simple and fast.

- Easy for practitioners to monitor.
- Cost-effective.
- Low risk of postoperative discomfort.

In addition, patients can, within reason, dictate the pace of treatment and see results relatively quickly.

Disadvantages

In contrast, the technique of tooth-bleaching is considered to have the following disadvantages:
- Active patient participation is required for home-bleaching. The drop-out rate from treatment can be as high as 50%. This draws into question how seriously concerned some patients are when requesting treatment to improve the appearance of their teeth, which serves as a warning if more destructive procedures are undertaken.
- Colour change is thought to be both dose- and time-dependent.
- The technique is open to abuse.
- A tray-based system can be a problem for patients who are prone to retching.

Clinical Technique

The clinical stages of the technique are as follows:
- Take a medical and dental history.
- Examine the soft tissues.
- Chart the dentition, noting the extent of any gingival recession.
- Ask about and test for sensitivity and record it.
- Record white spots areas on enamel and inform the patient, as these might get worse before they get better.
- Check the vitality of the teeth to be whitened and take radiographs where indicated clinically.
- Consider a diagnostic wax-up if combined treatments are proposed.
- Make a diagnosis and formulate a treatment plan.
- Normally one arch is bleached at a time, usually starting in the maxilla.
- The discoloured teeth to be bleached are agreed by the patient and dentist.
- Obtain informed consent. This must include a discussion of the benefits, risks, advantages, disadvantages, costs and the legal status of bleaching procedures. Be wary of promising a specific outcome and make sure patients understand their commitment to the procedure.

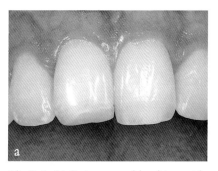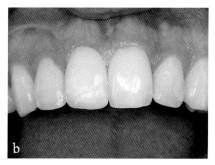

Fig 3-3 (a) Patient post-bleaching with an anterior restoration that requires replacement. (b) Patient with new incisal edge resin composite.

- Complete other treatment first, except anterior restorations (Fig 3-3). Fractured teeth or open cavities will need appropriate temporization. Warn the patient why you are doing this.
- Take an alginate impression.
- Complete a detailed laboratory prescription to produce a bleaching splint.
- In the laboratory the impression is cast in vacuum-mixed stone.
- Reservoirs can be provided. This is achieved by painting a thin coating of die relief, nail varnish or a separating agent over the labial surface of the teeth to be bleached (Fig 3-4). The finish line of the coating should be kept just below the gingival margin. The material acts as a space reservoir for the bleaching gel. There is some evidence that reservoirs confer no advantage to bleaching, and the decision about whether to include reservoirs rests with individual experience.
- The model is then trimmed to remove sharp edges. The base height of the cast should be trimmed so that the overall depth of the cast is as minimal as it can be. Casts with excessive height can cause the splint material to tear in the vacuum-forming machine.

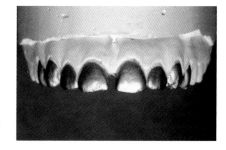

Fig 3-4 Block out resin placed to form reservoirs.

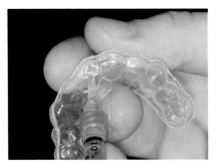
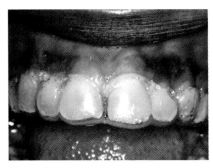

Fig 3-5 Bleaching gel being applied to the tray.

Fig 3-6 Tray loaded and in place.

- A thin 1mm polyvinyl sheet is vacuum formed over the model around the discoloured teeth.
- The splint should then be trimmed to 0.5–1mm below the gingival margin following the natural contour of the gingival margins. The sharp edges can be smoothed either with a rubber wheel or by gently using a flame gun along the edges.
- The tray should cover all occlusal surfaces but need not cover the palate. It is usually sufficient just to envelop the crowns of the teeth, as the retention of the splint is mainly gained from the bleaching gel being viscous rather than undercuts or coverage of the hard palate.
- Give the patient written instructions regarding care of the tray and application of the material (Figs 3-5 and 3-6). The tray can be cleaned with a toothbrush and toothpaste.
- The optimal amount of bleaching gel needed in the splints is small. Most manufacturers supply the gel in syringe form. Two syringes are more than sufficient to treat a single arch for a period of two weeks. It is normally convenient to supply a few syringes – typically three at a time – so that the patient needs to return for more if needed, as this allows the clinician to monitor closely the progress of treatment. If a patient is given an excessive number – for example, four or more syringes – it is possible that they might abuse the product. Currently manufacturers in the UK are not supplying instructions for patient use, so individual practices must therefore develop their own protocols.
- Reinforce the possibility of sensitivity.
- Dispense the bleaching material and advise that the splint is worn for six to eight hours, usually overnight. It is helpful to ask the patient to complete a diary sheet. The more often the bleach is applied the quicker

the process. Normally, a favourable outcome can be achieved within two weeks, but in some the process takes longer. This might reflect the severity of the discoloration or reduced patient compliance. Overcoming the latter is difficult and often an indicator of failure. If the patient fails to wear the splint as directed then the bleaching agent is in contact with the teeth for insufficient time and treatment fails. Frequent use and change of agent is the most effective regimen. Overnight bleaching was suggested initially for this technique but a better option, for some patients, is to wear the splint in the evenings and at weekends. Equally some patients are content to wear the splint during the day, but this can be more difficult if the patient works fulltime.

- Prescribe fluoride mouthwash for daily use.
- Arrange a review after one week with the proviso that the patient returns earlier if sensitivity proves to be a problem.

Review Appointments

It is recommended that the following routine is adopted at each review appointment:

- Examine the soft tissues for signs of inflammation, specifically trauma from the tray.
- Bleaching should be discontinued if severe sensitivity is being experienced.
- If sensitivity is increasing in severity, recommend bleaching on alternate days, perhaps using desensitising toothpaste in the splint on other days.
- Check shade against the original shade tab.
- Take photographs.
- Arrange review in a further week.
- Continue to review weekly.
- Explain to the patient that most of the bleaching change occurs in the first few hours and days after the bleaching has started and the shade is consolidated over the remaining period of treatment.
- When to stop treatment should be a joint decision made by both clinician and patient. Most simple cases are bleached within a few (usually two) weeks.
- Don't be tempted to discharge the patient until treatment is complete.
- It is advisable to overlighten slightly as there is usually some relapse.
- Reinforce that top-up treatments will be required.
- Record end-of-treatment shade and photograph.

Non-Vital Bleaching

Case Selection
Normally the cause of discoloration of non-vital teeth is the breakdown of blood products within dentine, which results in a darkened tooth. This process may occur soon after the loss of vitality but in other cases the process occurs over longer periods of time. Very dark teeth will take more time to whiten than mildly discoloured teeth. Therefore, for first-time users of this technique a mild to moderate stain will have a greater chance of achieving a successful outcome than a more intense one.

Very intense stains are difficult to manage. Non-vital bleaching is often not completely successful. The technique may have to be used in conjunction with a veneering technique or in extreme circumstances a full coverage indirect restoration such as a metal ceramic crown will be required. Because colour predictability can be difficult, a translucent all-ceramic crown may not be advisable, since the darkened tooth may still show through the crown and affect the ultimate shade of the restoration unless a system such as Procera has been used, which has an opaque alumina coping.

Sodium Perborate
Sodium perborate, as the name suggests, is another derivative of hydrogen peroxide, which breaks down in the presence of water to form sodium metaborate, hydrogen peroxide and nascent oxygen. This material has been used for years to bleach non-vital teeth using the "walking technique" – originally described by Nutting and Poe (1967), making sodium perborate the material of choice for bleaching non-vital teeth. Sodium perborate can also be mixed with hydrogen peroxide to potentiate the effect. The most cost-effective bleaching product for the bleaching of non-vital teeth therefore is a combination of 10 volumes or 3% hydrogen peroxide and sodium perborate mixed into slurry, which is not unlike wet sand. Both materials can usually be purchased through a local or hospital pharmacy. In theory heat can be used to increase the speed of reaction at the chairside. This is no longer indicated, however, and is positively contraindicated because of the potential for external root resorption.

Side-effects

The side-effects reported for non-vital bleaching are rare now that the walking technique has been adopted by a majority of practitioners. Previously, heat was used to activate the hydrogen peroxide, which increased the potential for heat to be transmitted to the surrounding gingival tissues. Where a temperature rise above 4°C occurs vital tissue can die, and a common consequence of this could be external root resorption.

Technique

The clinical stages of the technique are as follows:
- Obtain informed consent.
- Make radiographic assessments of the tooth/teeth to be treated specifically to exclude apical pathology and check the quality of the root canal treatment. If there is any doubt about the quality of the root canal therapy it is prudent to provide revision endodontic therapy before starting the bleaching procedure.
- Replace any defective restorations, which in some cases is often enough to improve the appearance of the tooth.
- Record baseline shade using a shade guide arranged in order of value.
- Isolate the tooth with rubber dam, which needs to be an effective seal. The seal of the rubber dam can be reinforced by the use of a rubber-a dam sealant. Remove all restorative material from the access cavity, paying special attention to remove any remaining restorative material from the labial walls of the access cavity, as it might be contributing to the darkness of the tooth.
- Refine the access and extend it to include the pulp horns. Any remaining darkened or stained dentine overlying the labial wall of the access chamber should also be removed with a bur. Care should be taken not to overdo this, as it might weaken the tooth.
- Remove gutta percha with a non end-cutting bur (for example, Gates Glidden, Dentsply Maillefer, France) to well below the gingival margin to allow space for a protective base overlying the gutta percha. This usually means that the gutta percha needs to be removed to at least 5mm down the radicular part of the root canal.
- Do not etch the access chamber as there is little evidence to suggest that acid etching before loading with the bleaching product confers any advantage; however, it takes very little time and may allow easier access for the bleaching agents.
- Place an inert base over the gutta percha to reduce the risk of the bleaching materials passing down to the apical tissues. Commonly used materials are zinc phosphate, traditional or resin-modified glass-ionomer cements or resin composites. The later materials are to be preferred, as they provide for a seal as well.
- Mix the sodium perborate with hydrogen peroxide to achieve a "wet sand" mix.

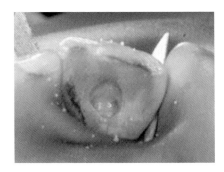

Fig 3-7 Sodium perborate in place.

- Place the mixture carefully over the base material and pack it against the labial wall of the tooth, leaving sufficient space for a small cotton wool pledget. For most endodontic procedures the size of the access cavity required to gain visible access to the root canal is of sufficient size for placing a slurry of hydrogen peroxide and sodium perborate into the tooth (Fig 3-7).
- Seal the access cavity with effective temporary cement – for example, zinc oxide and eugenol, IRM (Intermediate Restorative Material, Dentsply Ltd, UK) or a conventional glass-ionomer cement.
- Remove rubber dam.
- Emphasise to the patient that the procedure will take time. The patient should be reviewed at weekly intervals and treatment is completed when the colour change satisfies the patient's needs. At each review appointment the materials should be replaced with freshly mixed hydrogen peroxide and sodium perborate.
- Restore the access cavity with resin composite when the bleaching process is complete (Fig 3-8). To prevent further discoloration, it is important to seal the access cavity effectively. The preferred material for doing this is resin composite. It is sensible to use a light, more translucent shade further to lighten the tooth if this is required.

Advantages

The main advantage of the technique is that it is conservative of tooth tissue. However, equally important is the benefit of eliminating the need for a crown to restore the colour of the tooth, let alone the difficulties of providing a single crown to match the colour of the adjacent teeth successfully. Following root canal treatment, the strength of the tooth is frequently compromised. A

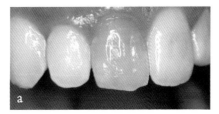 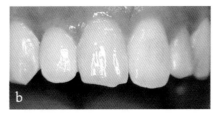

Fig 3-8 (a) Discoloured non-vital upper central incisor. (b) After non-vital tooth bleaching.

crown preparation will remove even more tooth tissue, possibly weakening the labial wall of the tooth to such an extent that it is lost and a post crown is needed to restore the tooth. The long-term prognosis of post-retained crowns is relatively poor. Bleaching non-vital teeth is therefore likely to prolong the life of the tooth by avoiding the need for a post-retained crown.

Side-effects

There is little potential for side-effects if the technique described above is followed. The most resistant part of the tooth to bleaching is often the gingival margin, possibly because insufficient gutta percha has been removed from the radicular part of the root canal or too much material has been placed to seal off the root-canal treatment. Or it may simply be that this part of the tooth is more resistant to bleaching. Either way it is often helpful to warn the patient of this potential problem before treatment is commenced. There is little potential for the bleaching procedure to weaken the tooth and increase the potential for fracture. The potential for fracture will largely depend on the size of the access chamber, which should always be kept as small as possible to allow good access for the endodontic procedures but large enough for the bleaching process.

Combination Techniques

Purchasing hydrogen peroxide in a concentration of 10 volumes from chemists or hospital pharmacists can sometimes be difficult. An alternative to sodium perborate is Bocasan (Oral B, Gillette Group, Isleworth, UK), which breaks down to form hydrogen peroxide and water. The concentration of hydrogen peroxide may be too low to brighten intensely darkened teeth. Therefore, practitioners may prefer other techniques. Carbamide peroxide, for example, can be used as a replacement for hydrogen peroxide and employed in a similar manner to that described above (say, for a walking bleaching technique).

Another variation is to bleach the tooth with the aid of a custom-made splint loaded with carbamide peroxide. This technique is probably easy to achieve because the materials are readily available to practitioners. As before, gutta percha is removed from the coronal third of the radicular canal to the same depth and a suitable base placed. The coronal/radicular base is required to protect the integrity of the root treatment providing for a coronal seal but an inter-appointment provisional material over the access chamber is not necessary. A vacuum-formed splint is used in the same way as for vital bleaching but, instead of sealing the material inside the pulp chamber, the access chamber is left unsealed. The vacuum-formed splint loaded labially and palatally can deliver the carbamide peroxide close to the tooth surface, so bleaching the tooth. The vacuum-formed splint should have a small reservoir made on the labial and palatal surface to limit the bleaching process to the single tooth. It is also helpful to cut back the splint on the adjacent teeth to ensure the bleaching gel cannot affect these teeth. Once the carbamide peroxide leaks into the saliva it is readily deactivated by enzymes.

In-Surgery Techniques

Carbamide peroxide (hydrogen peroxide) can be supplied in higher concentrations of 20-35% (6.6-11.5%) rather than the 10% (3.3%) used for home bleaching. The material is therefore caustic and, as a consequence, great care is needed when applying it in the mouth

Case Selection

Some patients request an immediate in-surgery result rather than a delayed outcome as achieved with the home techniques. The in-surgery techniques and materials achieve faster bleaching by using high concentrations of bleaching agent at the tooth surface with or without activation by light. In some patients a combination of in-surgery and home bleaching is helpful. It is important to realise that patients will respond differently and a combination of treatments may be appropriate. The in-surgery techniques have the advantage that the clinician has more control on the application than when relying on patient compliance. Chairside treatment time is, however, longer. A balance must therefore be achieved, and each case will be different. Arguably, the practitioner has less control over the final result than when a home-bleaching technique is used.

Clinical Stages

In-surgery techniques use concentrated carbamide peroxide or hydrogen peroxide, which have a potential to burn the soft tissues if contact occurs. The bleaching agent is applied to the surface for 15-30 minutes, either using a vacuum-formed splint similar to home bleaching or directly onto the discoloured teeth under rubber dam isolation used in conjunction with a dam sealer. Bleaching lights with turbo bleaching tips may be used to increase the rate of reaction of the carbamide peroxide. Whether this has any clinical significance remains to be demonstrated. Leakage around the edges of a splint should be carefully controlled when using a higher concentration, as the potential for damage to the soft tissues is much greater. Most techniques suggest 20-30 minutes as the maximum bleaching time at any one appointment, and a number of visits may be required to achieve the desired results.

Many clinicians use rubber dam to protect the gingival tissues if the material is to be applied directly. This is probably much safer than using other forms of moisture control. The split-dam technique is a compromise, which protects the lips and cheeks but not the gingival margins.

When in-surgery techniques and vital night-guard bleaching are compared, the following points are of importance:
- In-surgery bleaching treatment times can be lengthy and normally at least two visits are required.
- In-surgery bleaching with power lighting adds to chairside time and equipment costs, let alone practitioner time, significantly increasing the cost of treatment.
- For some patients the inconvenience of night-guard bleaching makes up for the procedure the more costly in-surgery.
- Safety concerns over burns to soft tissues have been expressed in relation to in-surgery techniques.
- It has been suggested that regression is quicker with in-surgery techniques compared with vital night-guard bleaching.
- Repeat treatments are as expensive as the initial treatments for in-surgery techniques.
- There is no clinical evidence that in-surgery techniques are more effective than vital night-guard bleaching.
- In-surgery techniques have some advantages over alternative techniques for the treatment of a single discoloured but vital tooth.
- There are reports of increased sensitivity when higher concentrations of carbamide peroxide are used.

Other Bleaching Techniques

Compared with a tray-based system, which can produce a shade change of seven shade tabs on the Vita shade guide, other bleaching techniques can produce an increase in value of 3–4 Vita shade tabs. In contrast with tray-based and in-surgery techniques these other bleaching systems can be purchased over the counter without the prescription of a dentist. The change in value is a somewhat slower process, with gradual increases in value noted in scientific studies. This change is often too subtle for the patient to fully appreciate and this could be considered a significant disadvantage of systems of this type. However, they probably have a place in the bleaching of already fairly white teeth (A3 or greater) or for top-up treatments between courses of vital night-guard bleaching or in-surgery techniques. It is important for practitioners, therefore, to be aware of the existence of these over-the-counter techniques and to have some knowledge of how they work.

Whitening Strips™
Whitening Strips™ (Proctor & Gamble, USA) were introduced to the US market in 2000. The strips are flexible polyethylene bleaching strips that are designed to deliver hydrogen peroxide in gel form directly to the labial surface of anterior teeth. The strips contain 6.5% hydrogen peroxide, and a two-week treatment period is typically recommended (Fig 3-9).

Topically Applied Systems
Recently a topically applied tooth-bleaching system in the form of a gel has been introduced in the US which contains 18% carbamide peroxide (Simply White, Colgate, USA). The system releases 6.03% hydrogen peroxide. It is applied with a special applicator to the labial surface of the teeth to be treated (Fig 3-10). The agent is applied twice a day for two weeks. Studies have shown that a two-week course of treatment can produce bleaching (increase in value) of 3–4 Vita shade tabs (Fig 3-11). The cost for a course of treatment is relatively low ($14.99/£ 8.25) and no significant side-effects have been reported. A European formulation has been developed and is currently being trialled.

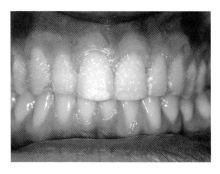

Fig 3-9 Whitening strips in place.

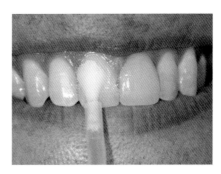

Fig 3-10 Topical whitening gel being applied.

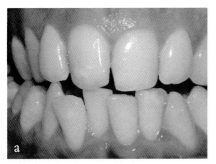
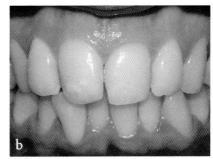

Fig 3-11 (a) Patient with discoloured teeth suitable for treatment with a topical whitening system. (b) After two weeks of topical tooth-whitening.

Whitening Toothpastes

Patient demand for whiter teeth is such that many toothpaste manufacturers have introduced whitening toothpastes to improve the brightness of teeth. In practice these agents are very effective at removing extrinsic staining, which can improve the overall appearance of teeth but not the underlying colour. This is of limited value, however, as extrinsic stain is more commonly found on the lingual aspects of teeth and is rarely a problem on the labial surface of teeth. Post-bleaching whitening toothpastes possibly do have a place in reducing and preventing the build-up of extrinsic stain, but their value in maintaining bleaching or whitening teeth is doubtful.

Microabrasion

The use of strong acids to remove stained enamel was first reported over 80 years ago. The technique is normally associated with the term "acid abrasion". It involves careful application of concentrated hydrochloric acid to a stained tooth. The major problems associated with this technique revolve around the dangers of using concentrated hydrochloric acid, albeit in a slurry, in the mouth. If mistakes occur and the acid is dropped onto either the oral soft tissues or the skin the result is burning that, if not treated immediately, can be disfiguring. For this reason the technique, although very effective, has not attained universal acceptance. Manufacturers have produced materials containing buffered acids and abrasives to remove the stain, and these are of more practical use to practitioners. Alternatively, localised reduction of the enamel with a tungsten carbide bur will often remove sufficient stain and, if necessary, a small resin composite restoration can be placed to mask the residual stain. The technique is particularly useful for localised "spots" rather than generalised discoloration.

Other indications for the technique include:
- Localised stains, typically found in fluorosis.
- Brown mottling rather than removal of white spots (Fig 3-12).
- Dark smoking stains but not those on incisal teeth where dentine has been exposed.

The technique is contraindicated for more generalised stains, such as tetracycline or age-related changes, which are best managed by means of vital bleaching.

Clinical Stages

The clinical stages for microabrasion are as follows:
- Apply rubber dam around the stained tooth or teeth, ensuring there is a good seal. A rubber-dam sealer can be used to improve the rubber-dam seal.
- Mix the concentrated hydrochloric acid with flour of pumice in a glass dappens pot to produce a consistency of wet sand.
- Alternatively use a proprietary premixed material. This is the authors' preference.
- Provide the patient with eye protection and a plastic bib to protect their clothing. Both the operator and the nurse also need effective eye and skin protection.
- Carefully apply the pumice and acid mixture onto the tooth surface using a flat plastic spatula and gradually agitate the material with a rubber cup. A speed-reducing handpiece can be used and care must be taken to avoid splattering of the material. The mixture effervesces and the colour of the tooth gradually changes. The technique is not usually successful after one

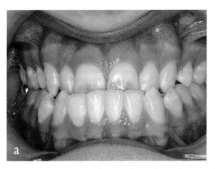 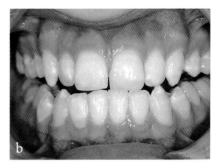

Fig 3-12 (a) Discoloured teeth with mottling. (b) After a combination of microabrasion and tooth-whitening.

application and may need repeated applications, but success is normally achieved in one half-hour appointment. Previously the tooth was pumiced between applications but this has been shown to be unnecessary.

- Wash the acid carefully away after each application under high volume aspiration – ensuring patient, nurse and clinician have eye protection.
- Continue the process until patient and clinician agree on the final colour.
- Note that a shallow depression is usually visible within the enamel after treatment has been completed. This is the result of the enamel removed by the acid.
- Fill the depression with an appropriately shaded resin composite, if required.
- Do not apply a fluoride varnish after treatment as the tooth quickly rehydrates. The patient should, however, avoid smoking and consuming those foods likely to cause stains – for example, curry, tea, coffee – for at least the first week following treatment.

Practitioners can find purchasing concentrated hydrochloric acid difficult. For this reason many clinicians suggest an enamel biopsy technique. The enamel biopsy technique, although similar in principle to microabrasion, is safer and more likely to achieve acceptance in general dental practice. In patients with fluorosis this technique can be helpful, as it removes localised stains, whereas for more generalised stains a vital bleaching technique would be more appropriate.

An enamel biopsy technique is carried out as follows:
- Remove (without rubber dam) the stained enamel surface with a high-speed water-cooled tungsten-carbide bur, with particular care being taken not to be overly destructive.

- Continue the process until the desired colour change has been achieved. Provided the biopsy or preparation does not involve dentine, a restoration is not usually required. Significant depressions in enamel will require restoration with resin composite. If a restoration is not placed it is helpful to apply a fluoride gel.
- Use a small localised resin composite restoration if dentine is exposed or the tooth becomes sensitive.

Further Reading

Dadoun MP, Bartlett DW. Safety issues when using carbamide peroxide to bleach vital teeth: a review of the literature. Eur J Prosthodont Rest Dent 2003;11:9-13.

Bartlett DW. Bleaching discoloured teeth. Dent Update 2001;28:14-18.

Bartlett DW, Walmsley AD. Home bleaching. Dent Update 1992;19:287-290.

Nutting EB, Poe GS. Chemical bleaching of discolored endodontically treated teeth. Dent Clin North Am 1967;Nov:655-662.

Chapter 4
Laminate Resin Composite Techniques

Aim

The aim of this chapter is to consider how laminate resin composite techniques can be used to provide aesthetic restorations for anterior teeth.

Outcome

On reading this chapter practitioners will become familiar with the materials and techniques best suited to improve the appearance of anterior teeth with laminate resin composite restorations.

Introduction

Resin composites have developed in tandem with dentine adhesive systems to the extent that resin composite adhesive systems can be used effectively to restore extensive defects in anterior teeth. Linking dentine-bonding agents and resin composites to enamel and dentine frequently removes the need for mechanical preparation. Caries removal and ensuring that the surface is clean and dry to maximise bond strength is all that is required for the restoration of many anterior teeth. This has considerable advantages for patients in that already damaged anterior teeth can be restored without further tooth preparation or the use of a laboratory to produce indirect restorations.

Current resin composites contain translucent enamel and dentine shades. Some manufacturers also provide opaquing or bleaching tooth shades, which are rarely needed. The resin composites are built up in a similar manner to making a porcelain crown in the laboratory (using core, dentine and enamel shades). The technique for these materials is not dissimilar to other direct build-up techniques, except that the majority of the build-up is done with dentine shades, with very little enamel shade used. A common mistake is to use too much of the enamel shades or the translucent shades, which can give a restoration that is very grey or blue.

Advantages of Directly Placed Resin Composites
The advantage of most porcelain laminate veneer techniques is minimal

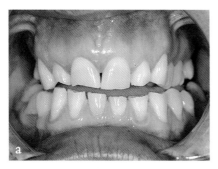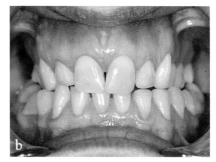

Fig 4-1 (a) Tooth wear with the patient in the retruded contact position (RCP). (b) Resin composite placed to restore the anterior teeth and stabilise the patient's RCP.

tooth preparation. The one limitation of this concept (especially on canines) is the potential to produce undercuts during tooth preparation relative to the path of insertion. Very bulbous canines, if minimally prepared, will have an undercut between the mesial and the distal surfaces. Alternatively, some clinicians advocate removing more tooth tissue to create space for porcelain and to remove the undercut, but that reduces the advantage of the technique being minimally invasive. Resin composite can be placed where it is needed and generally without tooth preparation (Fig 4-1).

Another advantage of direct resin composite veneers is the capacity to repair and refurbish the restoration over time. Minor fractures or localised staining or caries can be either removed or repaired with a resin composite used in conjunction with a dentine-bonding agent. It is useful when bonding old to new resin composite to use a silane-bonding agent to improve the bond between the two increments of material. Porcelain fractures can be repaired with resin composite but never look quite the same and, unless hydrofluoric acid is used, it is unlikely that a bond between the porcelain and the tooth or resin composite luting cement will be achieved.

Directly placed resin composite laminate restorations have another significant advantage in that the technique is very good for young (adolescent) patients not of an age to justify porcelain laminate veneers. Equally, directly placed resin composite laminate restorations are to be preferred when gingival maturation is not complete.

Disadvantages of Directly Placed Resin Composites
Probably the most significant disadvantage with directly placed resin com-

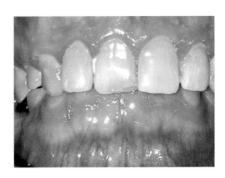

Fig 4-2 Excessive translucent resin composite has been placed to restore the incisal edge of tooth 11.

posites is the clinical time needed to produce an aesthetic result. Even though porcelain veneers involve a laboratory phase and consequently additional cost, it is the technician who spends the time shaping, contouring and colouring the restoration. The clinician need only lute the restoration into place. For some clinicians, the concept of a directly placed resin composite veneer is challenging and clinically satisfying, while for others this time is not well spent and they prefer the support of a technician.

Until recently, directly placed resin composite veneers lacked depth or variation in colour. Microhybrid resin composites overcome this to a large extent, but the clinical time needed to place these materials to good effect has increased significantly. More translucent enamel shade on the incisal tips can produce very acceptable results but can produce unacceptable ones if too much is used or they are used indiscriminately (Fig 4-2). Readers are referred to the Further Reading section for advice on selection of resin composites.

Clinical Techniques

Small and Moderately Sized Restorations
For the most part, using resin composites to restore anterior teeth is straightforward (Fig 4-3). There is little evidence to support the routine use of lining materials particularly as they effectively reduce the area available for bonding. The dentine-bonding agent will not only bond to the dentine and the enamel but also reduce the potential for microleakage by sealing the restoration tooth interface. Therefore, there is little need for a lining to protect the pulp from future damage.

Many manufacturers produce a series of enamel and dentine opacities or shades, usually based on the Vita system (Vita Zahnfabrik, Bad Säckingen,

45

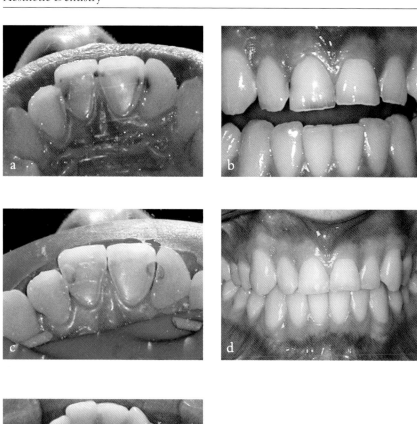

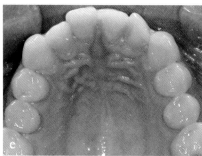

Fig 4-3 (a) Teeth suitable for direct build-up with resin composite featuring caries and tooth wear. (b) Unaesthetic anterior view due to tooth wear, resulting in translucent incisal edges. (c) Split rubber-dam isolation. (d) Completed treatment (anterior view). (e) Completed treatment (palatal view).

Germany). They effectively allow the clinician the opportunity to rebuild the broken-down tooth. The dentine shades replace the bulk of missing tooth tissue while the enamel replaces the more translucent surfaces. Some of these enamel shades are very translucent, and care should be taken not to over-use them, otherwise the restoration will appear too translucent or "blue". The use of these different opacities to rebuild the tooth means that the clinical technique of overbuilding the tooth to cut it down and then polish is not possible. The approximate shape and size of the tooth should be rebuilt, leaving only minor changes to the shape and a final polish. Overbuilding with the different opacities may result in the translucent shades being removed during the shaping and polishing stages.

Clinical Stages

- Prepare the tooth and remove peripheral caries, if present.
- Remove carefully pulpal caries, if present. There is little evidence that removing all the pulpal caries is necessary. Firm dentine is, however, required because soft dentine once sealed becomes harder and dryer and collapses, leaving a void under the restoration. In addition, the performance of modern adhesive systems on softened dentine is questionable. In most cases, provided the pulpal caries is reasonably hard, a well-sealed restoration will prevent further progress of the lesion.
- Ensure adequate moisture control. This can best be achieved with a rubber dam or judicious use of cotton wool rolls and salivary ejectors. Either way, it is essential to protect the preparation from contamination.
- Depending on the type of dentine-bonding agent used, either etch for 10 seconds or apply the first coat of the primer. Apply the second coat or the bonding agent to the tooth surface and agitate the material over the surface of the tooth for between 20-30 seconds, depending on the material.
- Place the preferred resin composite in increments and light cure according to the manufacturer's directions for use.
- Trim back any excess resin composite with a tungsten-carbide bur or a polishing diamond. Copy the surface contours of adjacent teeth to produce the shape of the restoration. If the margin approaches the gingival tissues position the bur to achieve the correct emergence angle between the restoration and the gingival tissues.
- Polish the resin composite with abrasive discs, rubber cups or flame-shaped finishing burs.
- Use a diamond polishing paste to achieve the final finished surface.

Changes to Shape and Size of Teeth

More extensive restorations as a result of either tooth wear or reshaping teeth – for example, closing diastemas – require different skills for building and maintaining the shape and colour of the tooth (Fig 4-4). Polyvinyl siloxane matrices can be particularly useful for rebuilding extensive restorations. These

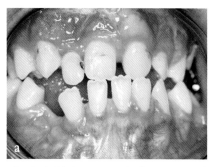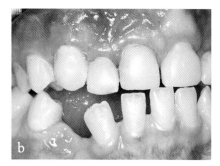

Fig 4-4 (a) Patient with diastemas and poor aesthetics. (b) Restoration with resin composite.

can be produced by taking an impression of the original tooth shape or, when this is not possible, from a diagnostic wax-up. This is useful in patients with tooth wear where the basic shape of the tooth has been worn away. The diagnostic wax-up is replicated by the matrix which is then used to support the build-up of resin composite.

Polishing

There are numerous techniques available, which include using discs and/or rotary polishing devices (Fig 4-5). There is little evidence that any technique is superior and much depends on the personal choice of the practitioner. Whatever technique is preferred, it is normal to use a reducing range of abrasives coupled with final finishing with a diamond polishing paste. There is a variety of shapes, from discs to cups and burs, all of which produce an effective result (Fig 4-6). Tungsten- carbide and diamond polishing points are particularly useful, as more abrasive ones can help shape the restoration before using the less abrasive polishing discs or cups.

Clinical Stages

- Plan the shape and colour of the restoration, possibly with a diagnostic wax-up.
- If using a diagnostic wax-up, copy the shape of the restorations with a polyvinyl siloxane matrix.
- Prepare the teeth. Some clinicians use bevels to improve the appearance and the bond. There is no clinical evidence to justify this step, so the decision whether or not to do so relies on clinical judgement. Essentially, a

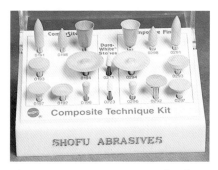

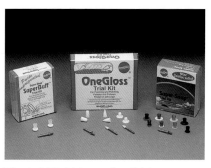

Fig 4-5 Resin composite finishing points.

Fig 4-6 Finishing and polishing systems for resin composite.

range of preparations (from virtually nothing to preparation similar to that required for a porcelain laminate veneer) will be required, depending on the specific needs of the case.

- Provided the clinician can achieve adequate moisture control, rubber dam need not be used. However, if moisture contamination cannot be avoided then rubber dam is essential.
- Apply the dentine-bonding agent according to the directions for use.
- If using a matrix, position it onto the palatal surfaces of the adjacent teeth.
- Incrementally build up the body of the restoration in resin composite. This is usually achieved with dentine shades. The incremental build-up is needed to overcome the polymerisation contraction of the material. This need not involve too many increments, normally three to four per restoration is sufficient, but will depend on the size of the preparation.
- Trim back and shape the excess with shaping burs or abrasive discs.
- Polish the restoration with finishing burs.
- Finally, polish the restoration with diamond polishing pastes.

Further Reading

Wilson NHF, Wilson MA. Indirect composite veneers. In: 1989 Dental Annual, Derrick Dentistry (ed). Guildford: Butterworth Scientific, 1989:268-272.

Chapter 5
Porcelain Laminate Techniques

Aim

Porcelain laminate veneer techniques have not been popular with certain practitioners, possibly because they have given poor results in comparison with those obtained by more traditional full-coverage techniques. The aim of this chapter is to reconsider porcelain laminate veneer restorations and consider how they can be used to good effect in modern-day aesthetic dentistry. The advantages of porcelain laminate veneers when compared to full-coverage techniques are also considered.

Outcome

On reading this chapter practitioners will be familiar with the indications, contraindications, advantages and disadvantages of porcelain laminate veneers along with the clinical techniques necessary to achieve optimal results with restorations of this type.

Introduction

The acid-etch technique was first described by Michael Buonocore in 1955. Rochette realised the potential of this for the micromechanical attachment of resin-based materials in 1973 and used the technique for the splinting of periodontally involved lower anterior teeth. Some ten years later porcelain-etching and the use of silane-coupling agents were concurrently described. The combined effects of these innovations have been that predictable outcomes for resin-bonded restorations are now possible for practitioners. These restorations can be bonded into place, which opens up opportunities for minimally interventive restorations (for example, porcelain laminate veneers).

Historical Perspective

Dr Charles Pincus first described Hollywood veneers in 1948. He used the technique to improve the appearance of teeth for actors and actresses, notably Shirley Temple. The veneers were held in place with denture adhesive and were removed after filming. Hollowed-out acrylic denture teeth, which failed, given a poor bond between the acrylic and resin composite, have been tried in the past. Similarly, preformed acrylic veneers marketed by Caulk in the 1980s tended to fail as a consequence of a poor bond between the acrylic and luting resin composite. Microfine resin composites have also been used, but these failed due to poor wear resistance, polymerisation shrinkage and inferior aesthetics with stain build-up. Porcelain veneers were first described in 1983 and introduced into the UK in 1984. Although porcelain is the material of choice, it should be noted that direct and indirect resin composite veneering techniques still have a place in the treatment of adolescent patients as intermediate restorations.

Indications

Porcelain laminate veneers are thought to be indicated in the following situations:
• Treatment of unsightly surface defects in essentially sound anterior teeth.
• Modifications to anterior tooth colour, shape, length and alignment.
• Restoration of fractured and endodontically treated anterior teeth.
• Treatment of anterior teeth with hypoplastic enamel.
• Masking discoloration caused by trauma, endodontic treatment, fluorosis and tetracycline staining (Fig 5-1).
• Repair of damage to anterior teeth, such as fractured incisal edges.
• Masking anatomical anomalies, including peg-shaped laterals (Fig 5-2).
• Treatment of amelogenesis imperfecta but not dentinogenesis imperfecta, as the enamel is prone to fracture off in the latter condition, leading to early failure of the restorations.

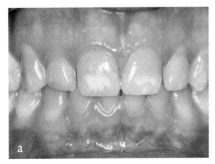 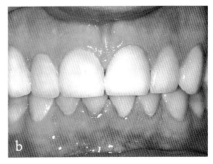

Fig 5-1 (a) Tetracycline staining. (b) Same patient with porcelain laminate veneers.

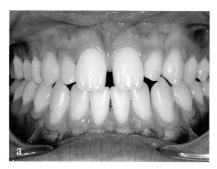 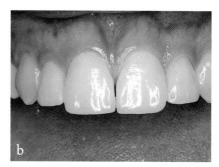

Fig 5-2 (a) Patient with a diastema and abnormally shaped lateral incisors. (b) Same patient with veneers in place.

- Closure of a median diastema, although this can be achieved quite easily with direct application of resin composite in carefully selected cases.

Contraindications

In contrast, porcelain laminate veneers are contraindicated in the following clinical situations:
- Poor oral hygiene.
- Where the restoration would have to have deeply placed subgingival margins.
- Atypical occlusal loading (for example, bruxism).
- Lack of adequate amounts of tooth tissue for bonding or poor-quality enamel, albeit in adequate amounts.
- Presence of large existing restorations, which favour a full coverage technique, as failure rates for porcelain laminate veneers placed on teeth with existing restorations are reported to be high.

Advantages

It is generally accepted that porcelain laminate veneers have the following advantages:
- Minimally interventive, especially when compared with full coverage restorations.
- Local analgesia is not normally required for tooth preparation or placement of the veneers.
- The aesthetic outcome can be exceptional.
- Typically no provisional restoration(s) are required.

Disadvantages

- Not a reversible technique, although previously thought to be, which is partly responsible for the confusion regarding the nature of preparation required.
- Relatively limited application, given that the tooth or teeth should be essentially intact.
- Technique sensitivity, in particular demanding preparation criteria and moisture control at placement.
- Long-term data are somewhat limited but encouraging — porcelain laminate veneers can reasonably be expected to last at least three years but clinical experience suggests that clinical service is typically in excess of five to 10 years.
- Possibility of marginal chipping and staining, especially if lute is exposed.

To Prepare or Not to Prepare?

When porcelain laminate veneers were first introduced into the UK, tooth preparation was not recommended. This was because practitioners were not sure how long porcelain laminate veneers would last and if they fell off the tooth would be back to square one. As a consequence, the technique was thought to be reversible. This had two effects: early retention rates were low because no tooth preparation had been carried out, and the effect on the emergence profile of the restored teeth was adverse, with marginal gingivitis adjacent to porcelain laminate veneers a common clinical finding (Fig 5-3). It has been shown that veneers placed without tooth preparation lead to an increase in associated periodontal problems (Fig 5-4).

Research has demonstrated that tooth preparation is therefore indicated. The advantages of tooth preparation are considered to include:
- Marked increase in bond strength to enamel when compared with non-preparation.
- Minimal effect on the emergence profile of the restored unit and, as a consequence, opportunity for excellent gingival response.
- Minimal, if any, increase in the overall dimensions of the tooth, facilitating an excellent aesthetic outcome and patient acceptance.

Tooth Preparation

Tooth preparation for porcelain laminate veneers can be broken down into the following stages:

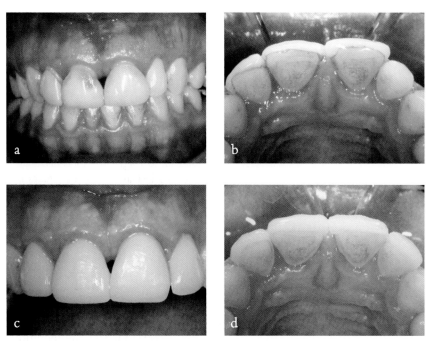

Fig 5-3 (a) Porcelain laminate veneers placed without preparation. This view is after a gingivectomy needed to remove the marginally inflamed gingival tissue. (b) Occlusal view showing how the veneers are bulky due to underpreparation. (c) Patient with new veneers. Note the black triangle and that of necessity the teeth are somewhat long. (d) Occlusal view showing how the veneers are less bulky and more anatomical.

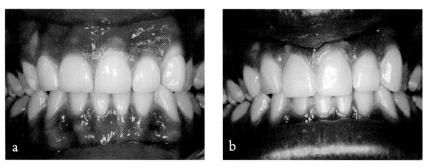

Fig 5-4 (a) Porcelain veneers placed in the patient's early teens prior to gingival maturation. The veneers have also been placed without preparation and are bulky. (b) Patient with new veneers. Note that tooth 14 has been disguised to look like tooth 13, which is missing.

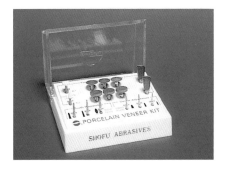

Fig 5-5 Veneer preparation kit.

- Typically, no local anaesthesia is required; prepare the tooth entirely within enamel. This is, however, very difficult; inevitably dentine will be exposed cervically during tooth preparation. This is not usually a problem in that patients rarely feel any discomfort. It does, however, mean that during luting procedures the use of a dentine-adhesive system is essential.
- A uniform labial reduction of 0.3 to 0.5mm (deeper in discoloured teeth and areas within individual teeth) is recommended. Studies have shown that depth of preparation is best controlled by using a depth gauge bur or a polyvinyl siloxane index.
- During tooth preparation it is important to reproduce the natural anatomical planes of the tooth. Typically, there are two to three planes in incisors and three or more planes in canines. Consequently, the bur should be angled to take account of this during tooth preparation. Special preparation kits are available (Fig 5-5).
- Chamfered juxtagingival or, wherever possible, supragingival cervical margins are recommended. Subgingival (> 0.5mm) margins may be considered to preclude the prescription of porcelain laminate veneers. In such cases a full-coverage restoration placed using a conventional luting technique may give the most favourable clinical outcome.
- Extend the preparation into but not through the proximal contacts. Some advocate preparing through the contact area – in particular, in areas where there are existing proximal restorations. If extension of the preparation to give a tooth/ceramic interface is not possible because of an existing restoration, a porcelain laminate veneer may be contraindicated.
- It is generally recommended that the incisal edge be reduced by 1mm and bevelled on the lingual or palatal surface (Fig 5-6). Recent studies have suggested, however, that porcelain laminate veneers placed with a feathered incisal edge have equivalent longevity to teeth reduced by 1mm to

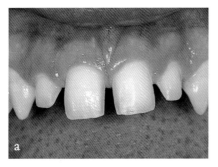 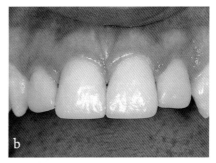

Fig 5-6 (a) Veneer preparations. (b) Patient with veneers placed.

give a bevelled incisal edge. It is suggested therefore that consideration be given to preparing a feathered incisal edge in selected cases.

- Overlapping, i.e. taking the preparation onto the lingual or palatal surface beyond the bevel, is recommended if the overall length of the tooth is being increased.
- Window preparations, which were originally recommended for canines to avoid altering canine guidance provided by the palatal surface and incisal tip, are no longer recommended. This is because it is difficult to create a perfect incisal margin and there is a high risk of enamel fracture with window preparations.
- Finally, the preparation is smoothed with fine-grade high-speed, water-cooled, diamond finishing burs. Any sharp line angles must be rounded.

Bur Selection

In terms of the burs to use for the gross and fine stages of tooth preparation, several of the bur manufactures have produced specific bur selections for this purpose, which frequently include matched finishing burs.

Other Clinical Procedures

Gingival retraction, using cords, is not usually necessary, as the margins are ideally placed supragingivally or juxtagingivally. If gingival retraction cord is necessary then a small-diameter (000) cord is recommended. To minimise the effect of the procedure on the periodontium it is important to optimise gingival health prior to commencing treatment. With atraumatic preparation techniques and good baseline gingival health, gingival control and haemorrhage are not usually problematic.

The use of an addition-cured polyvinyl siloxane or polyether impression material is recommended. The use of a special tray is rarely indicated, assuming good-quality stock trays are used. An impression of the opposing arch must be taken and sent to the laboratory. To register the occlusion it is suggested that a hard wax or a silicone interocclusal material is used. A face-bow transfer is required if the restorations are to be produced on a semi-adjustable articulator, which is strongly recommended if the incisal tips have been reduced. Shade-taking has already been covered in Chapter 2. Provisional restorations are not usually required, unless large amounts of dentine have been exposed during tooth preparation. Should this be the case, provisional restorations may be indicated. This being the case it is preferable to take an alginate impression before tooth preparation, which can then be used to produce provisional veneers. These can then be spot-etched and bonded into place. If a preoperative impression is not available, the prepared teeth can be built up to normal contour with carding wax and an alginate impression taken. Alternatively the teeth can be spot-etched and a resin composite material placed directly.

Luting Procedures

The luting of porcelain laminate veneers is very technique sensitive. To reduce the potential for error, the following is recommended:

- Do not try the porcelain laminate veneers on the model, as this will contaminate the fitting surface with die stone and reduce subsequent bond strength.
- Isolate tooth or teeth to receive the veneers with rubber dam. Special clamps are available that give good access to the gingival margins.
- Clean the tooth or teeth with oil-free slurry of pumice. The tooth can be left moist for try-in.
- Verify frosted appearance of restoration fitting surface and apply silane-coupling agent and allow to dry.
- Try in the restorations with a drop of water applied to the fitting surface. Do not try in the restorations dry as this will make shade assessment difficult. Some manufacturers supply water-soluble try-in pastes, which are particularly useful if some shade discrepancy exists between the preparation and the veneer. It has been shown that using a shaded try-in paste or water gives the best appreciation of the final shade of the restoration.
- Adjust fitting surfaces and proximal contacts of veneers one by one as required. Avoid excessive insertion forces, as this will fracture the restoration.

- Remove try-in paste with ethyl alcohol and if the fitting surface is contaminated re-etch with 37% orthophosphoric acid, which has been shown to be as effective as re-etching with hydrofluoric acid.
- Reapply silane-coupling agent.
- Etch tooth and apply dentine-bonding agent.
- Apply unfilled resin to restoration and tooth.
- Apply filled resin lute to the restoration and gently seat the veneer towards the gingival margin, rotating the veneer toward the labial surface of the preparation with a slight vibrating motion.
- Spot-cure the incisal edge for five seconds.
- Remove excess resin with a fresh brush, not cotton wool, as this drags the resin composite lute out of the marginal interface.
- Floss can be used to remove excess along the proximal margins.
- Cure fully, according to the manufacturer's directions for use. Usually each surface requires one minute of trans-tooth curing.

Finishing Procedures

- Should be minimal at the time of placement.
- Final finishing is best left until the next visit when the resin luting cement will be fully cured (at least 24 hours). This is because the silane bond requires 24 hours to mature fully.
- Use fine-grade (20mm) water-cooled diamond burs for fine finishing. A reciprocating handpiece with special finishing tips may be useful (Fig 5-7).
- Impregnated polishing tips are also useful.
- Additional finishing may be accomplished with finishing strips and discs, if required.

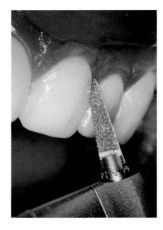

Fig 5-7 Profin™ tip and handpiece being used to remove resin cement excess.

- Fine diamond (0.5-0.7mm) polishing paste can be used for final finishing.
- Dental floss must pass interdentally and a probe must pass across the ceramic tooth interface without catching.
- Avoid overheating of the veneer during finishing, as excessive heat will fracture porcelain and degrade the bond or even injure the pulp. Water-cooling is therefore recommended.

Maintenance Procedures

- Staining at margins can be removed by refinishing with high-speed water-cooled diamonds.
- Small fractures can be ground out or repaired directly with resin composite (see Chapter 7).
- Significant fracture will require replacement of a veneer, but diagnose the reason for fracture before replacing the veneer.
- Persistent gingival inflammation, if mild, is best treated by refinishing of the margins and removal of excess bulk in the cervical third. If this fails, replacement of the veneer will be necessary

Further Reading

Brunton PA, Aminian A, Wilson NHF. Tooth preparation techniques for porcelain laminate veneers. Br Dent J 2000;189:260-262.

Brunton PA, Richmond S, Wilson NHF. Variations in the depth of preparations for porcelain laminate veneers. Eur J Prosthodont Rest Dent 1997;5:89-92.

Brunton PA, Wilson NHF. Preparations for porcelain laminate veneers in general dental practice. Br Dent J 1998;184:553-556.

Kreulen CM, Creugers NHJ, Meijering AC. Meta-analysis of anterior veneer restorations in clinical studies. J Dent 1998;26:345-353.

Chapter 6
Technical and Laboratory Considerations

Aim

Many of the factors that determine aesthetic success are dependent on close collaboration between the clinician and laboratory. Problems, as and when they occur, are generally a result of a breakdown in communication. The aim of this chapter is to examine in detail this important area of aesthetic dentistry.

Outcome

On reading this section practitioners will become familiar with the ways in which good aesthetic results are dependent on certain technical factors and vice versa. This understanding will improve the reader's ability to achieve optimal results.

Introduction

Optimising aesthetic outcomes for patients and operators depends on a variety of interrelated factors. These include the clinical–laboratory interface – in particular, colour communication and material selection, underpinned by appropriate tooth preparation and good-quality impressions. There is a range of ceramic materials available to practitioners today and this has led to considerable confusion. Choosing the right material needs careful consideration of the benefits of the material in terms of the potential aesthetic outcome and its physical properties balanced against the risks (for example, in terms of the amount of tooth tissue that requires removal). Equally, a discussion with the patient regarding cost and longevity is also required.

Having selected the material or materials that will be used, tooth reduction appropriate to the specific material or system must be carefully executed. Noting that both under- as well as over-preparation will affect the aesthetic outcome, it is important for practitioners to appreciate that different materials require subtly different tooth preparation. Research has shown that practitioners will frequently prepare a tooth in a way suitable for a gold inlay or onlay type restoration but request a resin composite or ceramic restoration to restore the unit. This is inappropriate, as gold is strong in thin section whereas resin composite and ceramic are not, and this poses a problem as resin composite will fracture off at the margins as a consequence of its relatively thin section.

Once measured, considered and appropriate tooth preparation has been carried out, of equal importance is how the integrity of the preparation and, not least, its relationship to the periodontal tissues are preserved. These are crucial to the long-term clinical outcome. Unfortunately adequate consideration to the temporisation of cases is rarely given. This frequently results in poorly contoured, leaking provisional crowns and bridges that encourage plaque accumulation and loss of pulp vitality in the long term. In addition to these points, practitioners often come to cement the definitive crowns to find that there has been recession or there is gingival haemorrhage to the extent that effective isolation for resin bonding procedures is well nigh impossible.

Technical Considerations for Full Coverage Restorations

Metal Ceramic Crowns

A metal ceramic crown unites two disparate materials, namely a metal alloy and porcelain. Both materials have markedly different physical and aesthetic properties. The success of this type of restoration relies on the strength of the underlying metal coupled with the aesthetic properties of the overlying porcelain. Of particular importance is the interface between the two materials.

The technician needs to mask the underlying non-reflective metal core with porcelain. This can be problematic. If this stage of the crown build-up process is not completed successfully, metal ceramic crowns can look very dark or, if over-opaqued, very high in value or "bright". To ensure that the aesthetics of the crown are optimal, the clinician needs to complete sufficient tooth reduction to create space for the different porcelains required to mask the underlying metal substructure. Insufficient space results in a crown with a relatively high proportion of core porcelain, which is bright, and so the crown appears to be too bright or too high a value. Appropriate preparation with sufficient tooth reduction provides the technician with the space necessary to build up an aesthetic crown of the same hue but with different chroma to provide depth to the colour of the crown, while still maintaining the labial contour of the tooth. The result is a natural-looking restoration. Under-preparation – in particular, in the cervical third – is a common occurance that results in a crown with a dark neck, given the lack of space for the technician to mask the underlying metal core effectively (Fig 6-1).

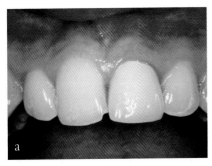
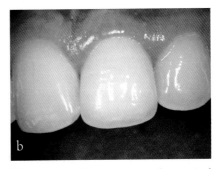

Fig 6-1 (a) Metal ceramic crown with insufficient depth of preparation in the cervical third. (b) After a Procera™ crown and resin composite addition to tooth 11. Note the excellent gingival response

All-Ceramic Crowns

With all-ceramic crowns there is no need to mask an underlying metal coping, as the restoration is metal free. As a consequence, all-ceramic crowns are increasing in popularity, offering good aesthetics and meeting patients' increasing demands for more biocompatible restorations (Fig 6-2). However, all-ceramic crowns have a limitation in that the strength of these restora-

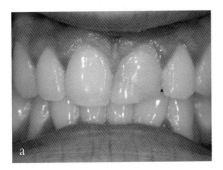
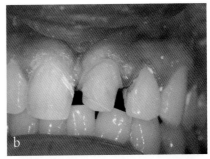

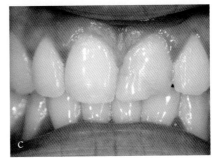

Fig 6-2 (a) Anterior teeth with resin composite build-ups. (b) Patient with the teeth and veneer prepared for Procera™ crowns. (c) Patient with the final crown and veneer in place.

tions is dependent on the strength of the core or coping used. Most copings or cores have a high value and are therefore comparatively bright. All-ceramic crowns require greater depth of preparation than metal ceramic crowns, as the practitioner must make room for the underlying coping and veneering porcelain. Exceptions to this are resin- or dentine bonded crowns and porcelain laminate veneers, which are made from feldspathic porcelain. Typically the depth of preparation is between 0.5–0.8mm for these restorations. As a consequence all-ceramic crowns cannot be described as minimal interventive techniques and in comparison with metal ceramic crowns are necessarily more destructive of tooth tissue. Systems that do not have opaque copings may not obscure the appearance of discoloured remaining tooth tissue or metal posts and cores. In these circumstances more tooth reduction may be needed to stop unwanted colours showing through the restoration. In certain cases the nature and depth of the discoloration may be such that an all-ceramic crown that does not have a coping is contraindicated.

Tooth Preparation

Teeth have a number of naturally occurring anatomical planes. These can be divided on the labial surface into a cervical/gingival, mid-labial and incisal. Removing the optimum amount of enamel and dentine in each dimension will give the technician just the right amount of space to make an aesthetic crown or veneer.

A useful tip is to make a matrix prior to commencing the preparation for a crown or veneer using an addition-cured polyvinyl siloxane putty. This matrix can additionally be used to produce provisional restorations, should this be required. When the operator believes that the preparation has been finished, divide the matrix through its mid-line (sagitally) using a scalpel. Replace the matrix over the prepared tooth and observe the amount of tooth reduced in all the planes along the labial and palatal walls, adjusting the preparation where necessary. Optimal labial reduction is 1.2–1.5mm for metal ceramic crowns, slightly deeper (1.5mm) for an all-ceramic crown and 0.5mm for a porcelain laminate veneer. It is not suggested that practitioners should routinely use a silicone matrix. It is, however, a useful technique for periodically checking and calibrating an individual practitioner's preparation technique.

If under-preparation leaves the technician with insufficient space on the buccal surface to produce a crown or veneer with a natural emergence profile, he or she must decide between achieving a matched buccal contour or over-

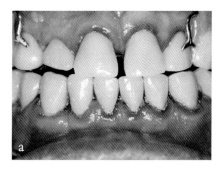
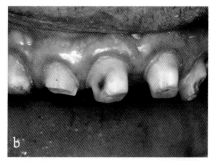
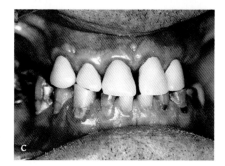

Fig 6-3 (a) Overbulked anterior crowns with marginal gingivitis. (b) Patient with refined preparations. (c) Diagnostic temporaries in place. Note resolution of marginal inflammation.

building the crown or veneer buccally to produce the right colour. Either way the result will be an unsatisfactory aesthetic outcome (Fig 6-3). Over-bulking the cervical third of crowns and laminate veneers can lead to plaque accumulation and problems with marginal inflammation, which may result in a less than optimal aesthetic outcome, in particular if the patient has a high smile line. Another area that is often under-prepared is the incisal half of the buccal or labial surface. Under-preparation may require the technician to move or widen the incisal edge to accommodate more porcelain, which would be needed to mask the underlying metal. In either situation, although under-preparation may seem more tooth friendly the converse can be true. In essence a balance must be struck between under- and over-preparation.

Stages of Tooth Preparation

The aim of tooth preparation is to provide sufficient space for the technician to make a crown or veneer which is both structurally durable and aesthetic. To achieve this effectively a practitioner must remove enough tooth tissue on the labial, palatal/lingual, incisal/occlusal and proximal surfaces to provide space for the crown without introducing undercuts, yet achieving a near-parallel preparation. Some clinicians prefer a staged process – for instance, occlusal/incisal reduction, then proximal reduction and then finally labial and palatal reduction, in that order.

It is suggested that practitioners proceed as follows:

- Design the crown – choose the material for the restoration. When choosing a material, it is helpful to consider the amount of preparation each type of material will require. A metal ceramic crown needs more labial/facial reduction than a resin- or dentine-bonded crown. An all-ceramic crown needs an equal amount of tooth reduction on the labial and palatal surfaces and is less conservative of tooth tissue than either resin- or dentine-bonded crowns or metal ceramic crowns.
- Assess and record the shade prior to tooth preparation.
- Test the vitality where indicated clinically and check the periapical status of the tooth radiographically.
- Local anaesthetic is given as appropriate.
- Obtain a preoperative matrix impression of the tooth or teeth which can be used to produce the provisional crown(s). Periodically take an additional one to check the amount of tooth reduction. Typically this is done with a polyvinyl siloxane or alginate impression, which is put to one side and used to make resin replica provisional crowns after preparation has been completed. It is recommended that if alginate is used it is not put in hypochlorite or wrapped in damp gauze, as excess moisture and, in particular, hypochlorite will retard the set of provisional crown and bridge materials.
- Another technique is to use modellers' wax (Fig 6-4) rather then polyvinyl siloxane or alginate. Softened pink wax is moulded around the tooth prior to tooth preparation and then allowed to cool and harden. Sufficient wax is needed to produce strength in bulk. The tooth is prepared and then a provisional crown and bridge resin is dispensed into the wax. The main advantage of the wax is that alterations to the shape of the crown can be readily achieved. For minimally prepared teeth some of the labial aspect of the wax can be removed labially to thicken the provisional crown, making them more durable.
- Cut grooves into the tooth to achieve the optimum depth for the crown preparation.
- Retention for crowns, irrespective of the type, is derived from the length of walls and angle of the preparation taper. Ideally, the taper should be around 15-20 degrees; less than this increases the potential for developing undercuts and greater taper reduces the retention of the crown. Most of the retention is obtained from the mesial and distal reduction.

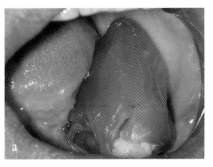 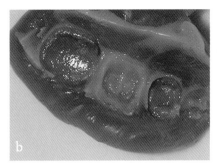

Fig 6-4 (a) Modellers' wax being adapted to a tooth to make a provisional crown. (b) Modellers' wax with provisional crown.

- Ensure that the proximal contact points are cleared.
- Follow the natural contour of the tooth.
- Check the occlusal reduction, in particular in relation to the occlusal contact area, ensuring that adequate space has been produced. It is also important to assess the depth of preparation in relation to excursive movements.
- Remove sharp-line angles and smooth the preparation. Typically this is done with fine-grade water-cooled finishing burs. Some clinicians find gingival margin trimmers and enamel chisels useful for refining the margins of crown preparations. Such instruments may be found to be especially useful for removing thin flashes of unsupported enamel.
- Place retraction cord if required. It is recommended that the cord is completely submerged in the crevice and left *in situ* for the impression and while provisional crowns are made.
- Make the provisional crowns, taking care to trim the margins appropriately. It is important to avoid any roughness and to ensure that each provisional crown has close marginal adaptation and should therefore seal the preparation margins.
- Take the impression.
- For most single units an occlusal record or facebow is unnecessary.
- Fit the provisional crowns using appropriate temporary cement. Typically, provisional crowns are cemented with zinc oxide eugenol temporary cement, which can be modified by the addition of a modifier paste. This is usually necessary when the preparations are very retentive and problems may be anticipated when it comes to removing provisional crowns. Modified temporary cement can also be very useful for the provisional cementation of

definitive restorations, which allows for ease of removal for modification if required prior to cementation using permanent cement.

It is important not to adopt a mechanistic approach to the preparation of teeth and, as such, it is not possible to be prescriptive about the shape of preparations. Each tooth is different, as is its relationship with the opposing dentition. Equally tooth wear may have already reduced the dimensions of a tooth. Practitioners should therefore focus on the principles of preparing teeth for crowns rather than mental images of the appearance of idealised preparations.

Central to the success of crowns is an understanding of the principles of retention – that is to say, what holds crowns in place. Generally speaking, a path of insertion that approaches the parallel is the most retentive. Shapes approaching pyramidal lines, with tapers around 45 degrees, are unretentive without using adhesive luting systems. It is inexcusable, however, to over-taper preparations in the mistaken belief that an adhesive luting system will compensate for poor technique. Conversely, lack of taper in a preparation increases the likelihood of introducing undercuts in the preparation. This is especially true of long preparations. The basic principles are the same for all types of preparation except for metal ceramics, where a deeper labial/facial reduction is needed to accommodate the combined thicknesses of metal and porcelain.

All-Ceramic Crowns

Patients are demanding more aesthetic, metal-free, biocompatible restorations. In response to this, manufacturers have produced systems capable of producing single-unit aesthetic metal-free restorations. Typically these are ceramic systems, with the exception of resin- or dentine-bonded crowns, which are made from feldspathic porcelains. There tends to be some confusion over the nature of current all-ceramic systems. These systems are broadly classified as follows:

- Computer-aided design/computer-aided manufacture (CAD/CAM) produced copings with veneer of conventional porcelain (Procera®).
- CAD/CAM without coping (Cerec®).
- Pressed ceramic (Empress I® and II®).
- Conventional build-up with alumina coping (In-Ceram® and Techceram®).

It is important to have an understanding of these ceramic systems. Special burs are available for tooth preparation for all-ceramic systems (Fig 6-5).

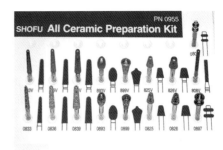

Fig 6-5 All-ceramic preparation kit.

CAD/CAM-Produced Coping with Conventional Build-up

Procera® (Nobel Biocare, Gothenborg, Sweden) is a relatively new system that also has an alumina coping. The die is scanned by a sapphire ruby laser to produce a digital image of the preparation and the image is sent by email to the "hub" laboratory. A computer-controlled milling machine uses the digital image to produce a core of densely sintered alumina which is then sent back to the originating laboratory. The core is then layered with conventional porcelains to produce the completed restoration. The coping can be produced in two levels of thickness (0.4 or 0.6mm), which will have an effect on the amount of dentine removed to provide space for the crown. The thinner coping allows the technique to be used in areas where space is limited and further tooth reduction is not possible. This might be, for example, in occlusal contact areas on teeth with short clinical crowns. The material can be adhesively bonded to teeth with Panavia® or cemented with more traditional cements such as glass-ionomer cements.

CAD/CAM without Coping

CAD/CAM systems use either an analogue crown to duplicate one in ceramic (Mikrona, Switzerland) or a digital impression of the preparation (Cerec®). Blocks of porcelain are milled to produce inlays or crowns, and both of these methods use conventional porcelains. Disadvantages of these systems include the relatively high cost of the laboratory equipment and that the restoration is largely limited to one shade only. This can restrict the quality of the aesthetic outcome achieved. Reservations have also been expressed about the fit of restorations produced in this way and also regarding the occlusal features of restorations made from a digital impression. Newer generations of these systems have largely overcome these limitations and further developments are to be expected – in particular, an increase in systems using optical impressions.

Pressed Ceramics

Examples of pressed glass ceramics are Empress I® or II® (Ivoclar Vivadent, Schaan, Liechtenstein). Empress I® is an all-ceramic pressed system and has the disadvantage that the restoration is made from one shade. In a similar way to Inceram®, Empress II® crowns and bridges comprise of two layers: an inner framework material made from lithium disilicate, coupled with an outer layer made from fluorapatite ceramic. The framework or core is made using the lost-wax technique. Wax is invested in a phosphate-bonded investment material and, after burn-out, the leucite-reinforced glass ceramic is pressed under pressure into the space left by the wax. Unlike Inceram®, the outer layer of Empress II® is thin. It is needed to improve the surface finish and characteristics rather than to make the crown's appearance acceptable. The fit surface of Empress I® and II® can be acid-etched with hydrofluoric acid allowing for adhesive bonding.

Conventional Build-up with Alumina Coping

Inceram® (Vita Zahnfabrik, Bad Säckingen, Germany) crowns consist of two distinct layers. The strength of the crown is derived from the inner core, which is made from zirconium and aluminium oxide; conventional porcelains are fired onto the core to produce the definitive restoration. To make an Inceram® restoration, fine alumina powder is applied to an absorbent refractory die, which is fired to produce a dense crystalline core structure. The core has a high strength and elastic modulus, but the improved strength is sacrificed at the expense of appearance, as the core material is very opaque. Conventional low-fusing porcelains are therefore applied over the core to create an aesthetically pleasing crown with high strength. Additionally, the high content of alumina makes it resistant to most acids and so a non-adhesive cement is used to cement the Inceram® crown.

Metal Ceramic Crowns

Metal ceramic crowns are made from a combination of a bonding alloy, which forms the metal framework onto which low- fusing porcelains are fired. A variety of alloys are available, together with many different porcelain systems. A variation in technique is Captek® (Schottlander and Davis, Letchworth, UK). Uniquely, this technique does not require a casting process to form the metal substructure, which can be an advantage for some laboratories and practitioners in terms of reduced costs and convenience. The basic structure of the crown is similar to conventional metal ceramic crowns, except that the core is made from a precious metal. A wax strip is applied to a refractory die and fired to produce a relatively porous surface, which is subsequently impregnated with a gold-rich wax strip. The combination is fired again and conventional porcelain finally applied to the resulting substructure. The crown is reported to have good marginal fit and biocompatibility. The crowns are considered to have a "warmer" appearance than conventional metal ceramic crowns because the yellow colour of the gold core pervades the crown. Until recently adhesive bonding of precious alloys to teeth was unreliable. The use of Panavia® resin luting cement, which bonds to yellow gold, has overcome this problem.

Provisional Crowns

Provisional crowns allow the practitioner to assess the shape and contour of the planned restorations. In addition the patient also has a chance to critique the shape, contour and fit of the final restoration before it is produced by the laboratory. This is very useful when major changes are planned to the anterior teeth – for example, an increase in overall tooth length or the closure of a midline or multiple diastema. There are essentially two ways of producing provisional crowns: the resin replica technique and the use of preformed crowns. The authors prefer the resin replica technique for the following reasons:

- Occlusal relationships are maintained and stabilised, as the provisional crown(s) have the same dimensions of the tooth prior to preparation, which can be more comfortable for the patient.
- Any reorganisation of the occlusion can be tested and adjustments made where needed before the definitive restorations are produced by the laboratory.
- Passive "over"-eruption of the opposing teeth, let alone movement of adjacent teeth, can be prevented.
- The gingival contour can be tested and adjustment carried out if needed to give an optimal emergence profile.
- Lower costs.
- A diagnostic wax-up can be duplicated and matched, allowing both the patient and dentist to test the shape, fit and potential success of the definitive restorations.

Preformed provisional crowns can achieve the same results as replica crowns. It is suggested, however, that the use of such crowns can be more time-consuming. In addition, preformed provisional crowns are not as accurate in terms of maintaining occlusal and proximal relationships.

Soft-Tissue Management

The aim of an impression is to record accurately the preparation including the margins to enable the technician to produce a well-fitting restoration.

Following preparation, the next stage is to make the provisional restoration and then take the impression, although some practitioners take the impression first. Whichever way round, an important part of impression-taking is management of the soft tissues.

The ideal position for the gingival margin is within the gingival crevice. The need to use gingival retraction techniques in such situations is questionable. In these circumstances the impression material should record the margin adequately, provided there is no bleeding. If bleeding is a problem some practitioners may use astringents to reduce it. A recent innovation is a material called Expa-syl™ (Kerr/Hawes UK, Peterborough, UK). This material uses a paste containing aluminium chloride, which acts as an astringent to control bleeding, and micronised kaolin and water, which act as a barrier. The material is left in the gingival sulcus for one to two minutes and then washed away before the impression is taken. Expa-syl™ is useful for preparations finished within or just below the level of the gingival cervice, otherwise retraction cord is more appropriate (Fig 6-6).

Some practitioners use electrosurgery for minor alterations to the gingival contours. An advantage of this technique is that it can control haemorrhage in traumatised gingival tissues. Care must be taken when using this equipment, as inappropriate use may cause tissue death. Following electrosurgery, the impression can be taken immediately or after a few days to allow the tissues to heal. A delay is advantageous, as recession is relatively common following electrosurgery. Electrosurgery is contraindicated in patients with pacemakers, and plastic instruments must be used to reduce the risk of electric shock to the operator.

The most commonly used method of soft-tissue management is retraction cord used with or without an astringent. Techniques vary from a single cord, which is removed as the impression material is syringed around the preparation, to a dual cord approach with one left in and one removed. The authors' preference is to leave the cord in while taking the impression. With very deep margins a number of questions are raised. First, should the tooth be crowned? Should a direct restorative material be left beneath the crown? Or should crown-lengthening be used to expose the margin? Each clinical situation is different and for this difficult clinical dilemma there is no easy answer.

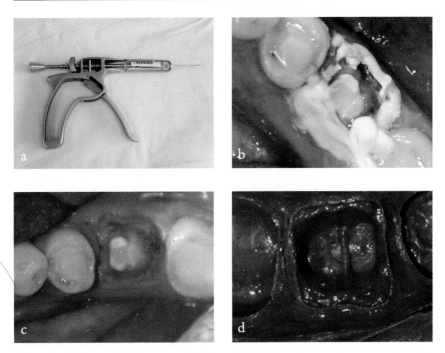

Fig 6-6 (a) Expa-Syl™ system. (b) Expa-Syl™ placed around a preparation. (c) Expa-Syl™ washed away, showing preparation margins of tooth. (d) Impression of the preparation.

Impression Materials

Essentially there are four types of impression materials available to practitioners. These are:
- polysulfide
- polyether
- condensation-cured polyvinyl siloxane
- addition-cured polyvinyl siloxane.

Polysulfide-based impression materials are not used routinely because of the long setting time and poor accuracy. In contrast, condensation-cured polyvinyl siloxane impression materials are used more widely, despite their poor dimensional accuracy related to shrinkage. There is clear evidence, however, that practitioners should use either an addition-cured polyvinyl siloxane or a polyether impression material, preferably dispensed by an automixing machine.

Polyether impression materials are used mostly for implant cases because of their rigidity, which precludes their use when significant undercuts are present. If polyether materials are used, care must be taken when the impression is disinfected. The impression can absorb water, and this will cause distortion. Consequently the impression must be transported dry.

Clinical Stages for the Resin Replica Technique

Conformative Approach
When no changes are planned to the patient's occlusal scheme, the stages needed to produce a provisional crown using the resin replica technique are:
- Take an alginate impression of the arch, including the teeth to be prepared. A helpful tip if resin- or dentine-bonded crowns are planned is to add material to the teeth to be prepared on the labial surface to increase the bulk of the crown(s). This is because a preparation depth of 0.5mm results in a resin replica crown which is too thin to withstand occlusal loading and the temporary cement will be seen through the crown, which appears very "white". This technique is also very useful when provisional veneers are necessary.
- Put the alginate impression to one side. Do not place it in a disinfection solution of hypochlorite, as this will retard the set of provisional crown and bridge materials. Equally, it is important to keep the impression damp,, but excessive moisture will retard the set.
- Take the shade at this stage.
- Carry out tooth preparation.
- Place retraction cord if needed, totally submerging the cord in the crevice.
- Take the impression, leaving the retraction cord in place.
- Check that the preoperative alginate matrix can be reseated.
- Mix the provisional crown and bridge material and place it in the matrix impression, taking care not to introduce air blows. Try not to place excessive amounts of material, as the crown(s) or bridgework will require excessive finishing.
- Reseat the matrix and allow the provisional crown and bridge material to set to a gel stage.
- Remove the alginate impression. The provisional crown(s) or bridgework will either come out with the matrix or stay *in situ*. If the temporaries are still in the alginate, it is possible and often easier to trim the margins with a scalpel. If the temporaries are retained on the teeth, it is necessary to remove them from the preparations before full set of the material locks them on to the prepared teeth by engaging proximal undercuts.
- Excess material should be removed with high-speed water-cooled fine-grade finishing burs and finishing discs.

- If there are air blows in the provisional crowns these can be rectified by applying light-cured resin composite of a suitable shade, provided the air blows are not at the margins of the crown. If there are significant numbers of air blows, the air blow is large or located at the restoration margin, then it is prudent to start again.
- Retry the crowns and check the occlusion and marginal adaptation.
- The crown(s) or bridgework is then cemented with an appropriate temporary cement. Traditionally, it has always been considered that eugenol-containing temporary cements are contraindicated if resin-bonded restorations are planned. This is because eugenol is retained in the dentinal tubules, resulting in plastinisation of the monomer and subsequent softening and discoloration of the resin composite luting cement. However, recent investigations have shown that the routine use of an etchant on dentine will remove residual eugenol from the dentinal tubules. So it is now possible to use eugenol-containing temporary cements for the cementation of provisional restorations of preparations destined to be restored with a resin-bonded restorations.
- Check the occlusion with articulating paper. The most commonly used articulating paper is around 40-50μm thick (Bausch Articulating Papers Inc., One Chestnut Street, Nashua, NH 03060, USA). Provided it is used carefully, listening to the teeth contacting, it is perfectly acceptable. Other papers can be much thinner – GHM paper at 10-15μm thick – with the most accurate being Shimstock (Hanel Medizinal, Nurtingen, Germany), which is 10μm thick or less. Whichever technique is used, the view of the patient and their perception of contacts is most important. It is recommended that Miller forceps are used to hold articulating paper. It also very helpful to check centric contacts with one colour of articulating paper and excursive contacts with another colour paper. With the conformative approach minimal occlusal adjustment is typically required.
- Instruct the patient to return if there any problems – particularly if the provisional crown(s) become uncemented. The patient should also be warned about eating high-colour-content food.

Reorganised Approach

This is when changes are planned to a patient's occlusion – for example, an increase in the vertical dimension of the occlusion. The stages to producing resin replica crowns or bridgework in such cases are as follows:

- Take upper and lower alginate impressions.
- Use a facebow to record the position of the upper arch in relation to the terminal hinge axis.
- Record centric relation or the retruded contact position with a suitable

material. A hard wax (for example, Moyco Beauty Wax) or hard silicone bite-registration paste is recommended.

- Ask the laboratory to mount the casts on a semi-adjustable articulator.
- Adjust the vertical dimension of occlusion and ask the laboratory to diagnostically wax-up your planned occlusal and aesthetic scheme (Fig 6-7).
- Ask the laboratory to do this in tooth-coloured wax and show it to the patient to get their agreement to what is proposed. Take and agree the shade at this point.
- Ask the laboratory to duplicate the cast and diagnostic wax-up, once it has been agreed, in vacuum-mixed stone and ask them to provide a blow-down template. Some laboratories will send a vacuum-formed soft splint. This is not suitable, as the material is too thick and fine detail will not be reproduced. A material with a thickness of 1mm is considered to be optimal.
- Alternatively, if directly placed resin composite restorations are being used to restore worn anterior teeth, a polyvinyl siloxane template can be made on the duplicated cast at the chairside using an addition-cured polyvinyl siloxane impression putty.
- Carry out tooth preparation. With multiple preparations this is sometimes done in stages.
- At this stage it is possible to proceed directly to the impression stage. Alternatively, provisional crown(s) and or bridgework can be placed to assess the patient's response to the proposed occlusal and aesthetic scheme. This latter approach is strongly recommended if multiple teeth have been prepared and substantial occlusal changes are planned. It is disastrous to proceed to the definitive stage and then find that either the patient cannot tolerate the change or does not like the appearance of the completed crowns and bridges.

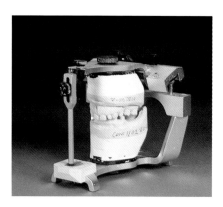

Fig 6-7 Diagnostic wax-up on a semi-adjustable articulator.

If proceeding directly to the impression stage, the clinical stages are as follows:
- Place retraction cord if needed, totally submerging the cord in the crevice.
- Take the impression with an appropriate impression material.
- Mix the provisional crown and bridge material and place it in the template, taking care not to introduce air blows. Try not to place excessive amounts of material, as the crown(s) or bridgework will require excessive finishing.
- Reseat the template and allow the material to set to a gel stage.
- Remove the template. The provisional crown(s) or bridgework will either come out with the template or be retained on the prepared teeth. If the temporaries are still in the template it is very easy to remove them by gently flexing the template. If the temporaries remain on the teeth it is helpful to remove them from the preparations before they are fully set, as the material can lock into undercuts.
- Excess material can be removed with finishing burs or discs.
- The crown(s) or bridgework is then cemented with an appropriate temporary cement.
- Check the occlusion with articulating paper with ideally a thickness of 10-15μm. Miller forceps can be used to hold the paper. It is helpful to check centric contacts with one colour of articulating paper and excursive contacts with another colour paper.
- Instruct the patient to return if there are any problems – particularly if the provisional crown(s) become uncemented. The patient should also be warned about eating high-colour-content food.

If the provisional restorations are to be placed to test tolerance and patient acceptance it is suggested that the clinical stages are as follows:
- Provisional crown and bridge material in various Vita® shades are now available. This is helpful if the provisional restorations are to be in place for some time. Patients must be warned, however, that any provisional crown and bridge material will pick up staining from certain heavily coloured food stuffs – curries, for example. This is particularly relevant if the provisional crowns are to be in place for some time.
- Mix the provisional crown and bridge material and place it in the template, taking care not to introduce air blows. Try not to place excessive amounts of material, as the crown(s) or bridgework will require extra finishing.
- Reseat the template and allow the material to set to a gel stage.
- Remove the template. The provisional crown(s) or bridgework will either come out with the template or be retained on the prepared teeth. If the temporaries are still in the template it is very easy to remove them by gently flexing the template. If the temporaries are still *in situ* it is helpful to

remove them from the preparations before they are fully set, as the material can lock into undercuts.

- Excess material can be removed with finishing burs or discs.
- The crown(s) or bridgework are then cemented with an appropriate provisional cement.
- Check the occlusion.

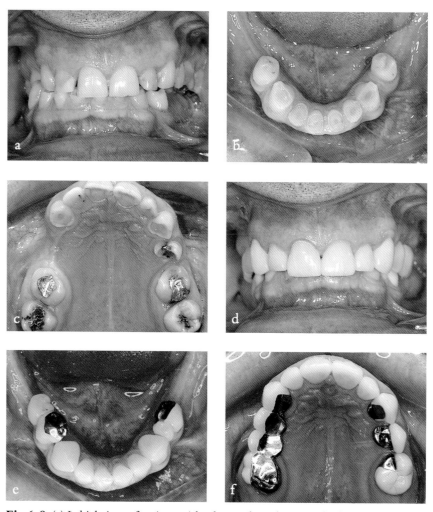

Fig 6-8 (a) Labial view of patient with advanced toothwear, which requires a reorganised approach. (b) Lower arch. (c) Upper arch. (d) Labial view of patient post-treatment. (e) Lower arch of patient post-treatment. (f) Upper arch of patient post-treatment.

- Review the patient, adjusting the occlusion, contour and shape of the crowns if necessary.
- Check the patient is happy with the proposed changes.
- Take alginate impressions of both arches.
- Take a facebow record to allow the maxillary cast to be mounted in a semi-adjustable articulator.
- Record centric relation or the retruded contact position using a hard wax and ask the laboratory to mount the lower cast using this record.
- The laboratory can then produce a customised anterior guidance table on the articulator, which can then be used to copy the guidance to the definitive crowns.
- Equally, an index can be made of the provisional crowns, which records the shape and contours of the planned restorations. The technician can use this alone or in tandem with the customised anterior guidance table to produce definitive crown(s) or bridgework that mirror the planned restorations (Fig 6-8).

Further Reading

Brunton PA, Smith P, McCord JF, Wilson NHF. Procera all ceramic crowns: a new approach to an old problem? Br Dent J 1999;186:430-434.

Brunton PA. Preparing anterior teeth for indirect restorations. Dent Update 2004;31:131-136.

McDonald A. Preparation guidelines for full and partial coverage ceramic restorations. Dent Update 2001;28:84-90.

Chapter 7
Aesthetic Compromises and Dilemmas

Aim

Success is a poor teacher. We learn a great deal from our mistakes. The aim of this section is to consider aesthetic compromises and dilemmas and in doing so prevent less than optimal outcomes.

Outcome

On reading this section practitioners will be able to prevent aesthetic compromises and deal effectively with common aesthetic dilemmas.

Introduction

One thing certain in restorative dentistry is that all interventions and treatments, however well done, are ultimately likely to fail. Long-term failure is to be expected, and practitioners should be able to give an indication of the longevity of restorations. Arguably, without this information the consent process is not informed. Central to our understanding of aesthetic failures is that treatment can be well executed technically, yet the patient can deem it a failure for aesthetic reasons alone. It is important, therefore, to consider failures, and more importantly to judge how to foresee and prevent them. Various pitfalls and dilemmas with the aesthetics of anterior restorations will be considered.

Informed Consent

Essential to the consent process is a discussion of alternative procedures and a comparison of the risks, costs and benefits of the various options. Bear in mind that aesthetic dentistry is something that patients generally request rather than something they need. This is in contrast to dental treatment needed to secure oral health. Consequently, doing nothing is also a treatment option that must be both considered and discussed. It is helpful to outline alternative treatments for the management of unsightly anterior teeth in terms of increasing levels of intervention, outlining the risks, costs and benefits (Fig 7-1). If bleaching is a

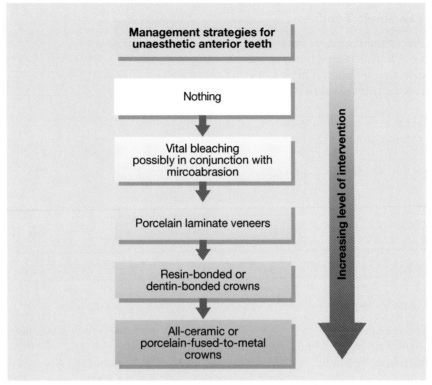

Fig 7-1 Management strategies for unaesthetic anterior teeth.

possible treatment option then central to the consent for bleaching procedures at the present time is informing the patient of the current legal status of bleaching. Without this information the consent is not informed.

With aesthetic procedures it is important that what the patient requests and what treatment you can deliver are one and the same. Problems arise when this is not the case. Patients may attend seeking unrealistic treatments. Following a discussion as to what is possible, a course of action should be agreed and informed consent obtained. A written treatment plan should also be provided to the patient at this stage. Crucial to this process is an acceptance and understanding by the patient of what you have both agreed, — that is to say, what the treatment outcomes will be. If there is any doubt about this it might be prudent to decline to treat such patients.

The Single Tooth

Practitioners are not infrequently faced with the problem of a patient with a single discoloured or damaged tooth requesting treatment to improve their dental appearance. This is a difficult clinical scenario to manage effectively, especially if the tooth is intact.

Treatment options for a single discoloured tooth include:
• doing nothing
• bleaching
• microabrasion, if appropriate, with or without bleaching
• crowning or veneering the tooth.

Doing Nothing

Doing nothing is seldom an option when the patient has specifically requested treatment. However, it is important not to agree to provide treatment that is out of your range of skills and experience and you consider will have little, if any, chance of success or will be detrimental to the patient.

Bleaching

If the tooth is non-vital, management is relatively straightforward using a non-vital bleaching technique. If the tooth is vital and structurally sound, then a vital bleaching technique may be indicated. A modified bleaching technique is used in that carbamide peroxide is placed in the splint which may or may not have a reservoir, with the splint sectioned or cut away from the adjacent teeth. The cut-away limits the extent to which bleaching gel changes the colour of the adjacent teeth. This will usually work, but it is difficult to limit the whitening to the affected tooth. It is probably better to whiten the discoloured tooth and then whiten the entire arch, if appropriate, to compensate for collateral bleaching of adjacent teeth. If bleaching of the entire arch is not appropriate, a more controlled way of treating a single discoloured tooth is to use an in-surgery technique, accepting the limitations of this technique.

Microabrasion With and Without Bleaching

Microabrasion can be a useful technique for localised superficial discolorations. Localised discolorations affecting a single tooth that could be amenable to microabrasion are rare. The technique can be supplemented with in-surgery or night-guard vital bleaching as appropriate.

Crowning or Veneering the Tooth

Crowning possibly best treats the single discoloured tooth, including

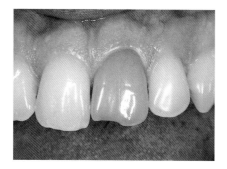

Fig 7-2 Discoloured tooth that has failed to whiten with non-vital bleaching. This tooth will need either a veneer or, more correctly due its discoloration, a crown with a coping of either metal or ceramic.

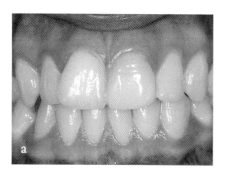
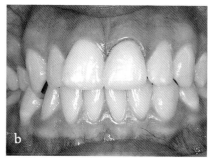

Fig 7-3 (a) Patient with a single veneer on 21; the patient is unhappy with the appearance. (b) Replacement veneer for the patient illustrating how difficult it is to match one veneer.

extensive restorations. Discoloured sound teeth that have failed to respond to bleaching or have an atypical shape may best be managed with a porcelain laminate veneer (Fig 7-2). The difficulty with single-unit aesthetic restorations is that it is almost impossible to match them successfully to adjacent sound teeth. Consequently it is preferable to treat pairs of anterior teeth with indirect restorations. This might mean an adjacent sound tooth being prepared, which flies in the face of a minimally interventive approach. To mitigate the effects of this a combination of a crown and veneer may be used (Fig 7-3). It is important in this situation that the patient understands why two teeth rather than one tooth need to be prepared.

Porcelain Laminate Veneers

Porcelain laminate veneers may be found to perform well in clinical service over a number of years if case selection, tooth preparation and placement techniques are optimal. Inevitably, all restorations, whatever their type, can deteriorate in clinical service. Central to remedying problems is an understanding of why the failure has occurred. Simply replacing the restoration will almost certainly result in a repeat failure, which will damage your confidence in the technique and your patient's confidence in you. The various types of failure that can occur with porcelain laminate veneers are considered here, and the remedial action necessary either to repair the restoration or to ensure success with a replacement restoration is discussed. It is important to note that many of the failures that occur with porcelain laminate veneers may also occur with resin- or dentine-bonded crowns. The treatment required to remedy the fault is similar in most cases .

General Failure During Clinical Service
There is an increased incidence of failure of porcelain laminate veneers in teeth with (large) existing restorations. This occurs particularly when any existing restorations, notably proximal resin composite restorations, are not completely covered by the veneer. Extensive restorations require a hybrid-type preparation or, preferably, a complete coverage technique.

Loss of resin-luting cement can lead to catches, marginal staining, interfacial leakage and possibly caries that can be difficult to diagnose in its early stages. Equally, poor preparation technique can lead to problems with the emergence profile of the restoration. This can facilitate plaque accumulation, leading to a recalcitrant marginal gingivitis, which is difficult to resolve – not to mention poor anterior aesthetics.

Complete Loss
Complete loss of a porcelain laminate veneer may occur as a result of the following reasons:
- Error in the use of the silane coupling agent; typically applying insufficient silane coupling agent – failure is likely to occur soon after cementation.
- Improper wetting of the laminate by the resin-luting composite, possibly subsequent to contamination of the fitting surface during, for example, placement of the porcelain laminate veneers on the stone die to check the fit.
- Movement of laminates when the resin-luting cement is at a gel stage.
- Resin-based tints or luting cements exposed to the surgery lights for extended periods of time, prior to placement of the laminate. This is a relatively common problem with modern-day high-intensity operating lights.
- Improper acid etch. This can be difficult to assess; however, the following may be useful guide:
  - satin appearance – under-etched

- ▪ frosted appearance – proper etch
- ▪ chalky appearance – over-etched
- Parafunctional habit or atypical occlusal loading.
- Trauma can result in complete loss of a laminate veneer restoration.

Marginal Inflammation

Chronic inflammation of the adjacent gingival tissues will result in poor aesthetics, notably in patients with a high smile line. Gingival inflammation associated with porcelain laminate veneers may be the result of one or several of the following factors:

- Poor finishing techniques leaving residual positive or negative discrepancies. This can commonly occur when a low-viscosity resin luting cement has been used. It is especially easy to leave an excess of resin-luting cement inadvertently .
- Placing laminates subgingivally even with excellent finishing techniques will usually cause some gingival inflammation, let alone invite other difficulties at the impression and placement stages, notably achieving good moisture control. Matters are further complicated if the margin is on dentine or cementum.
- Inadequate or inappropriate oral hygiene.

Remedial treatment involves replacing the laminates or refinishing the margins subsequent to concerted action to minimise the inflammation.

Bulky Laminates

With adequate tooth preparation a porcelain laminate veneer restoration should reproduce the original contours of the tooth. Failure to do so can result in overbuilt or bulky laminate veneers, which the patient may find hard to tolerate (Fig 7-4). Bulky laminate veneers can be due to the following:

- Inaccurate placement at the cementation stage. This is most likely to happen when the tooth has been inadequately prepared and there is a lack of a positive seat during cementation as a consequence.
- Use of too much resin composite luting cement, which should be approximately 0.1mm thick after seating.
- Laminate design is too thick. Ideally, the body of the laminate should be approximately 0.4mm thick and at the margins approximately 0.1mm thick. Frequently the technician has to bulk the tooth out due to inadequate preparation.
- Incorrect trimming and finishing of laminate in the laboratory.
- Replacement laminates placed without complete removal of the original restoration along with the luting cement.

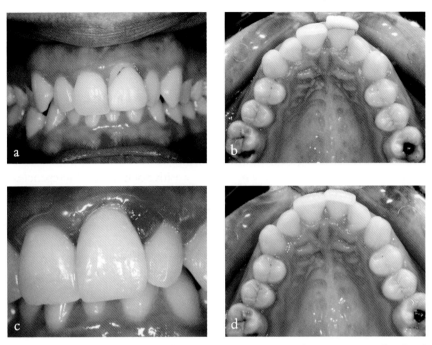

Fig 7-4 (a) Bulky laminate with poor margins. Note inflammation on the distal aspect. (b) Occlusal view emphasising the incisal bulk. (c) New porcelain laminate veneer with improved emergence profile. (d) Occlusal view of patient post-treatment shows improved contour.

Remedial treatment for bulky laminates is to replace the restoration.

Peeling of Laminate

If the laminate veneer starts to "peel" at the margins this is can be due to one of the following:

- Margins not sealed at placement stage.
- Ledging related to improper laminate adaptation or excessive resin luting cement, which should be approximately 0.1mm thick when the restoration is seated.
- Layer of bonding agent — that is to say, unfilled resin — is too thick and there has been cohesive crack propagation in this layer of the adhesive system.
- Improper seating of the laminate at the cementation stage, possibly as a consequence of binding at the proximal contacts.

Remedial treatment is the replacement of the porcelain laminate veneer.

White Flecks Under Laminate Surface

White flecks can affect the aesthetic outcome of laminate veneer restorations. They are usually due to one of the following:

- A void in the resin luting cement layer, which is due to too much pressure having been applied to the laminate during placement. Excessive pressure means that the resin composite cannot flow normally and a "rebound effect" occurs, typically often at the margins.
- Improper or excessive placement of opaquers.

Remedial treatment for a white fleck is to replace the laminate restoration.

Marginal Staining

The trend toward supra- or juxtagingival preparation margins for laminate veneers increases the likelihood of the margins being visible. Consequently, staining around the marginal interface of the restoration compromises the aesthetics. This can, of course, be compounded by the use of dual or chemically cured resin-composite luting cements. Staining or discoloration of the marginal interface may occur as a result of the following:

- Veneer is too bulky at margins and not closely adapted, which allows staining of exposed resin-composite lute by more-than-average tea or coffee drinking.
- Incomplete finishing of the margins leaving a resin composite "rim". This commonly occurs when using low-viscosity luting cements.
- Poor oral hygiene and care of laminates.

Remedial treatment includes instructing the patient on laminate care (for example, proper brushing and flossing). Light refinishing of margins with fine-grade water-cooled high-speed diamond burs may be required to remove excess lute and refurbish the existing interface. Dual- or chemically cured resin composite luting cements containing a tertiary amine as chemical initiator may discolour over time. This can result in both marginal staining and darkening of a laminate as the underlying luting cement discolours.

Incisal Angle or Edge Fracture

If this occurs, it is usually a consequence of poor case assessment and rarely a technical deficiency in the restoration. As a general rule, fracture soon after placement is likely to be a consequence of poor occlusal management. In contrast, fracture after many years of service is probably as a result of stress fatigue. Other causes of incisal angle fracture include:

- Atypical occlusal loading.
- Parafunctional habits (for example, nail biting).
- Veneer does not "wrap around".
- Veneer finished at labial incisal line angle.
- Patient applies excessive biting forces during the initial 24-hour period immediately after placement.

Small fractures can be repaired with resin composite. The other option is to replace the laminate. If an occlusal problem is suspected it is prudent to make the replacement with the aid of a semi-adjustable articulator and the maxillary cast mounted with the aid of a facebow and programmed with centric and protrusive occlusal records.

Resin-Composite Laminate Techniques

Indirectly placed resin-composite veneers are rarely used today because of the success of directly placed aesthetic resin composites. Directly or indirectly placed resin-composite laminate veneers have certain specific problems in clinical service. These are as follows:
- Staining of the entire laminate.
- Wear of the labial surface.

Staining of Entire Laminate
This only occurs when the laminate veneer has been made of resin composite. Remedial treatment includes refinishing or refurbishing the restoration or remaking the laminate using porcelain or ceramic.

Wear of the Labial Surface
Wear tends to be a feature of laminate veneers made of resin composite. It occurs as a consequence of one or a combination of the following:
- Use of extremely abrasive dentifrice or a hard toothbrush.
- Overzealous or too frequent toothbrushing.

Remedial treatment would include remaking the laminate restoration using porcelain or ceramic or simply the addition of an increment of resin composite to effect a repair.

Fracture of Crowns and Bridgework

When a patient presents with fracture of anterior crown or bridgework, it is important to diagnose the reason for failure before considering the various

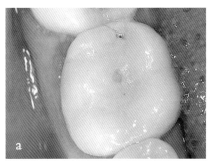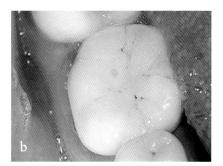

Fig 7-5 (a) Inadequate occlusal reduction leading to fracture of an all-ceramic crown. (b) New all-ceramic crown for the patient using a thinner Procera® coping.

treatment options. Fracture of the unit or units, particularly soon after cementation, is probably because of excessive occlusal loading. Fracture of the restoration after years of clinical service is likely to be a consequence of stress fatigue of the material or trauma. The treatment for a fracture of an anterior crown or bridge is usually confined to the following:

- Direct restoration of the defect, most commonly with suitably shaded resin-composite restorative material placed with the aid of an adhesive system. This is normally a short- to medium-term repair, as a replacement is inevitable.
- Larger fractures will require restoration replacement.

Prevention of fracture of crowns and bridgework is best achieved by:

- Assessing the patient's occlusion at restoration placement to include the use of articulating paper at the preparation and finishing stages.
- Not placing preparation margins in static or dynamic occlusal contact areas.
- Adequate occlusal reduction in occlusal contact areas (Fig 7-5a).
- Selection of an appropriate material where there is atypical occlusal loading (Fig 7-5b).

Intraoral Repair of Fractured Crowns and Bridgework
Fractures of the porcelain or ceramic of crowns or bridgework have until recently been very difficult to repair. Repairs were frequently short-lived and ultimately the restoration required replacement to guarantee a predictable aesthetic result. The advent of newer, more predictable adhesive systems, intraoral conditioning treatments (etching and sandblasting) for porcelain, ceramic and metal coupled with resins that adhere to metal and silanised porcelain or ceramic have changed this. The newer techniques and

materials now offer practitioners the possibility of predictable intraoral repair of fractured crowns and bridgework.

Before deciding whether to repair a fractured crown or bridge it is important to consider the following:

- **Clinical condition of the bridge:** A repair should only be undertaken when the bridge or crown is clinically satisfactory in all other respects. Leaking margins, catastrophic fracture of the bridge and/or secondary caries will typically dictate that the bridge or crown is replaced.

- **Occlusal factors:** This is of particular importance when a patient presents with fractured porcelain or ceramic, which is frequently suggestive of an occlusal interference during protrusive and lateral excursions. These are often overlooked when the occlusion is checked prior to cementation, with only centric occlusal stops checked and adjusted. It is strongly recommended that both centric and excursive occlusal contacts are checked and adjusted appropriately at the time of placement, and this should prevent subsequent fracture of the porcelain or ceramic. Equally, following repair the occlusion should be checked carefully.

- **Time to fracture from cementation:** As a general rule fracture soon after cementation is likely to be due to an occlusal problem. Fracture after a long period of use is usually suggestive of stress fatigue failure.

- **Fractured portion available:** If the fractured piece of porcelain or ceramic is available it can be bonded back into place, using a suitable bonding agent, after being etched and coated with a silane-coupling agent.

- **Nature of the fracture site:** If the intraoral fracture site is predominately metal a bonding agent with a special affinity for metal, such as a 4-META type of resin, will be required. Commonly, a resin opaquer will also be required – in particular, when a lighter shade of resin composite is needed for the repair. If the fracture site is predominately porcelain or ceramic with a small amount of metal exposed then intraoral etching of the porcelain or ceramic will be sufficient to retain the resin composite repair.

- **Extent of the fracture:** Minimal fractures of porcelain or ceramic are more amenable to repair with resin composite, while more extensive fractures will usually require replacement of the bridgework or crown. Other methods to affect an aesthetic repair of more extensive bridgework porcelain fractures include preparation of the fractured tooth while leaving the bridgework in place, for either a porcelain laminate veneer or another metal ceramic crown.

- **History of previous fracture:** It is suggested that repeat failure of a previously repaired bridge or crown is better treated with a replacement crown or bridge after the reason for repeated failure has been diagnosed.

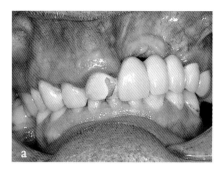

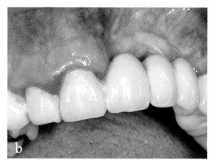

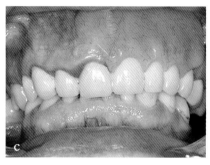

Fig 7-6 (a) Porcelain fractured from upper right one (11). (b) Post-op view following repair with Cojet™. (c) Gingival veneer in place.

Repair Materials

A variety of bridge repair kits are available to the practitioner. These products commonly include the following:

- Either hydrofluoric acid (9.5%) or acidulated phosphate fluoride (1.23%) for intraoral etching of porcelain.
- A silane-coupling agent.
- A metal bonding agent (for example, a 4-META type resin).
- An opaque resin to obscure underlying metalwork if required.
- An unfilled resin.
- A midway-filled densified resin composite for the ultimate repair.

Cojet™ (3M ESPE UK Ltd), a novel material, has been introduced for the management of fractured resin composite and ceramic restorations (Fig 7-6a). This versatile system does not require an intraoral etchant material and has additional uses, namely pretreatment of resin composite, ceramic and metal restorations prior to cementation with a resin-luting cement. The system revolves around silicatised sand, which can be used both intra- and extra-orally to pretreat resin-composite, ceramic and metal surfaces. The sand (aluminium oxide), particle size 30μm, which is coated with silicone dioxide, is placed in a mini-sandblaster under pressure (2-3 bar, 30-42 psi) and the fracture site treated for 15 seconds. The particles of sand hit the surface with a very high impact energy, which mechanically roughens the surface. The high energy generated causes the silicone dioxide particles to melt and become incorporated "tribochemically anchored" into the substrate surface up to a depth of 15μm while the sand particles are aspirated away. Subsequent application of a silane-coupling agent to this modified surface allows the attachment of a resin composite luting cement or restorative material (Fig 7-6b,c). The various stages for using this material to repair restorations are illustrated in Table 7-1.

Table 7-1 **Procedure for repairing fractured porcelain and metal-ceramic restorations with Cojet™ (3M ESPE)**

Porcelain restoration	Metal-ceramic restoration
1. Apply rubber dam.	
2. Patient and operator should wear safety glasses.	
3. Sandblast (Cojet™ sand) the ceramic to be repaired for 15 seconds.	3. Sandblast the ceramic to be repaired for 15 seconds.
4. Silanate for 30 seconds and air-dry.	4. Silanate for 30 seconds and air-dry.
5. Apply unfilled resin and light-cure for 20 seconds.	5. Cover the metal with opaquer and light-cure for 10 seconds.
6. Incrementally apply a resin composite and light-cure for 40 seconds.	6. Apply unfilled resin and light-cure for 20 seconds.
7. Finish with microfine high-speed water-cooled burs.	7. Incrementally apply a resin composite and light-cure for for 40 seconds.
	8. Finish with microfine high-speed water-cooled burs.

Further Reading

Robbins JW. Intraoral repair of the fractured porcelain restoration. Operat Dent 1998;23:203-207.

Appendix

Suggested Materials

Preparation Burs
- All-ceramic preparation kit Shofu™
- Veneer preparation kit Shofu™
- Composite technique kit Shofu™

Resin Composites
- Optident™ Enamel Plus HFO
- Coltene Whaledent™ Miris
- Heraeus Kulzer™ Venus
- Dentsply™ Esthet X
- Kerr™ Point 4

Resin Composite Finishing Systems
- 3M ESPE™ Soflex Discs
- Dentsply™ Enhance finishing and polishing system
- Shofu™ One Gloss
- Dentsply™ Prisma Gloss

Bleaching Products
- Optident™ Opalescence (10% carbamide peroxide)
- Oral B™ Bocasan

Other Products
- 3MESPE™ Cojet Bridge Repair Kit
- Dentsply™ Calibra Resin Luting System
- Optident™ Opalustre Microabrasion System
- Moyco™ Beauty Wax

Impression Materials
- 3MESPE™ Impregum
- 3MESPE™ Dimension Addition Cured Silicone
- Dentsply™ Aquasil Ultra

Composite Luting Cements
- Kuraray's Panavia F
- Dentsply™ Calibra
- Ivoclar™ Variolink
- Kerr™ Nexus 2

Index

Index

Single tooth 83
Smoking 20
Sodium perborate 32
Soft-tissue management 71
Surface topography 14

T

Technical and laboratory
  considerations 61
Tetracycline staining 27
Tooth preparation 61, 64
Tooth size 1
Tooth wear 12
Trauma 20

U

Urea peroxide 23

V

Value 11
Veneers 22
Vital night-guard bleaching 37
Vital teeth 19

W

Whitening toothpastes 21, 39
White spots 28

Quintessentials for General Dental Practitioners Series

in 36 volumes

Editor-in-Chief: Professor Nairn H F Wilson

The Quintessentials for General Dental Practitioners Series covers basic principles and key issues in all aspects of modern dental medicine. Each book can be read as a stand-alone volume or in conjunction with other books in the series.

Publication date,
approximately

Oral Surgery and Oral Medicine, Editor: John G Meechan

Practical Dental Local Anaesthesia	available
Practical Oral Medicine	available
Practical Conscious Sedation	available
Practical Surgical Dentistry	Autumn 2005

Imaging, Editor: Keith Horner

Interpreting Dental Radiographs	available
Panoramic Radiology	Autumn 2005
Twenty-first Century Dental Imaging	Spring 2006

Periodontology, Editor: Iain L C Chapple

Understanding Periodontal Diseases: Assessment and Diagnostic Procedures in Practice	available
Decision-Making for the Periodontal Team	available
Successful Periodontal Therapy – A Non-Surgical Approach	available
Periodontal Management of Children, Adolescents and Young Adults	available
Periodontal Medicine: A Window on the Body	Autumn 2005

Implantology, Editor: Lloyd J Searson

Implantology in General Dental Practice	available
Managing Orofacial Pain in Practice	Spring 2006

Endodontics, Editor: John M Whitworth

Rational Root Canal Treatment in Practice	available
Managing Endodontic Failure in Practice	available
Managing Dental Trauma in Practice	Autumn 2005
Preventing Pulpal Injury in Practice	Autumn 2005

Prosthodontics, Editor: P Finbarr Allen

Teeth for Life for Older Adults	available
Complete Dentures – from Planning to Problem Solving	available
Removable Partial Dentures	available
Fixed Prosthodontics in Dental Practice	available
Occlusion: A Theoretical and Team Approach	Spring 2006

Operative Dentistry, Editor: Paul A Brunton

Decision-Making in Operative Dentistry	available
Aesthetic Dentistry	available
Indirect Restorations	Spring 2006
Communicating in Dental Practice: Stress Free Dentistry and Improved Patient Care	Spring 2006
Applied Dental Materials in Operative Dentistry	Spring 2006

Paediatric Dentistry/Orthodontics, Editor: Marie Therese Hosey

Child Taming: How to Cope with Children in Dental Practice	available
Paediatric Cariology	available
Treatment Planning for the Developing Dentition	Autumn 2005

General Dentistry and Practice Management, Editor: Raj Rattan

The Business of Dentistry	available
Risk Management	available
Practice Management for the Dental Team	Autumn 2005
Quality Matters: From Clinical Care to Customer Service	Autumn 2005
Dental Practice Design	Spring 2006
IT in Dentistry: A Working Manual	Spring 2006

Quintessence Publishing Co. Ltd., London